Leprosy

MEDICINE IN THE TROPICS SERIES

Tropical venereology (Second edition)
O. P. Arya   A. O. Osoba   F. J. Bennett

Practical epidemiology (Third edition)
D. J. P. Barker

Diagnostic pathways in clinical medicine (Second edition)
B. J. Essex

Recent advances in tropical medicine
H. M. Gilles

Leprosy
R. C. Hastings

Tropical microbiology
D. G. Montefiore   K. O. Alausa   O. Tomori

Trypanosomiasis
B. A. Newton

Epidemiology and the community control of disease in warm climate countries
(Second edition)
D. Robinson

Medicine in the tropics (Second edition)
A. M. Woodruff   S. G. Wright

Leprosy

Anthony Bryceson MD FRCP
Consultant Physician,
Hospital for Tropical Diseases, London, UK

Roy E. Pfaltzgraff MD DSc(Hon)
Medical Consultant,
American Leprosy Missions Inc.,
Elmwood Park, New Jersey, USA

THIRD EDITION

CHURCHILL LIVINGSTONE
EDINBURGH LONDON MELBOURNE AND NEW YORK 1990

CHURCHILL LIVINGSTONE
Medical Division of Longman Group UK Limited

Distributed in the United States of America by
Churchill Livingstone Inc., 1560 Broadway,
New York, N.Y. 10036 and by associated companies,
branches and representatives throughout the world.

First edition 1973
Second edition 1979
Third edition 1990

First edition published under the title
Leprosy for Students of Medicine by
A. Bryceson and R. E. Pfaltzgraff.

ISBN 0-443-03373-0

British Library Cataloguing in Publication Data
Bryceson, Anthony D. M.
  Leprosy. — 3rd. ed.
  1. Man. Leprosy
  I. Title   II. Pfaltzgraff, Roy E. (Edward) III.
  Series
  616.9′98

Library of Congress Cataloging in Publication Data
Bryceson, Anthony.
  Leprosy/Anthony D. M. Bryceson, Roy E. Pfaltzgraff. — 3rd ed. p.   cm. —
    (Medicine in the tropics series)
  Includes bibliographies and index.
  1. Leprosy. I. Pfaltzgraff, Roy E. (Roy Edward) II. Title. III. Series:
Medicine in the tropics.
  [DNLM: 1. Leprosy.   WC 335 B916L]
  RC154.B83   1989
  616.9′98–dc20

Produced by Longman Singapore Publishers (Pte) Ltd.
Printed in Singapore

Preface to the third edition

In the 11 years since the second edition, leprosy has become increasingly respectable as a subject of research and many more scientists have come to join the ever-faithful band of field workers.

Great strides have been made in the immunology and chemotherapy of leprosy which have altered concepts of epidemiology and control. Animal models of leprosy have added materially to our knowledge of the transmission of leprosy. These five chapters have been extensively revised and a new chapter added on *Mycobacterium leprae* itself: despite problems with its culture (nearly solved as we go to press) there is now much information of its physiology, biochemistry and antigenicity that is essential for an understanding of the disease. There is also a better understanding of the physical and psychological disabilities endured by leprosy patients. The stigma of the disease, however, remains fully entrenched in many parts of the world, and still separates patients with leprosy from their fellows.

Sadly, the same years have seen the death of many great leprologists of the older generation, and of the younger too, including Ayele Belehu, M. Christian, F. Davey, R. Guinto, A. B. A. Karat, S. G. Browne, R. Cochrane, H. Heikeshoven, C. V. Lara, J. C. Pedley, C. C. Shepherd and B. D. Molesworth. We salute them all.

Although we have expanded the lists for further reading, our aim is still to provide a basic knowledge and explanation of leprosy for students in developing countries and for doctors and scientists elsewhere who want an introduction to the disease and the problems it continues to pose.

Once more we are indebted to Mr Ray Phillips at the Middlesex Hospital, London, for his painstaking care with the plates and we thank Mrs Annie Urqhart and Mr John Garbera for drawing the figures. We are also grateful to Dr A. C. McDougall for Plate 4, to Dr Margaret Brand for Figures 11.2–11.4, Dr D. L. Leiker for

Figure 5.7, Dr Tom Rea for Figure 8.7, St John's Hospital for Diseases of the Skin for Figures 4.24 and 8.3, Mr Peter Cheese for Figure 12.5, to Professor V. Møller-Christensen for permission to publish Figure 3.7, to John Wright & Sons for permission to reproduce Figure 10.5, to the Editors of Bulletin of the World Health Organisation for Figures 14.1 and 14.2, to the Editor of International Journal of Leprosy from which Figures 2.2, 4.28 and 7.2 are adapted, to the Editor of Leprosy Review for Figures 16.2, 16.3 and 16.4, and to Churchill Livingstone for Figure 14.2. Dr M. J. Colston and Dr Indira Nath kindly commented on Chapters 2 and 7 respectively; any errors or omissions are our own. The colour plates are printed by courtesy of Pharmanova, a division of Scanpharm, Denmark. Ulla Bryceson indexed all three editions.

London and New Jersey, 1990   A.B.
                                                               R.E.P.

From the preface to the first edition

This book is born of a course which we run at Garkida for medical students of Ahmadu Bello University. During the course we try to teach the principles of the basic disciplines involved in a study of leprosy, as well as the clinical and social aspects of the care of patients. We have tried to do the same thing here, which makes the presentation of some chapters a little unusual, and we have done our best to distinguish proven fact from accepted dogma and speculation, but it has not always been possible to reconcile the enormous clinical experience of yesterday with the newer concepts about leprosy which are emerging today.

Although our experience is mainly African we hope that this book may fill a gap elsewhere too, and that it may be of use to doctors in the field as well as to the students for whom it is written.

1973   A.B.
                                                           R.E.P.

To our wives, Ulla and Violet, whose mixture of tolerance and encouragement has run to three editions.

Contents

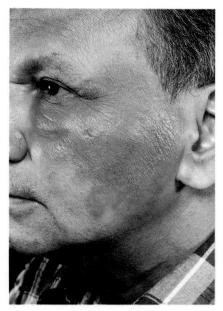

Plate 1 Plaque of borderline tubercloid leprosy in an Indian, showing the copper colour that may be seen in lesions in pale skins.

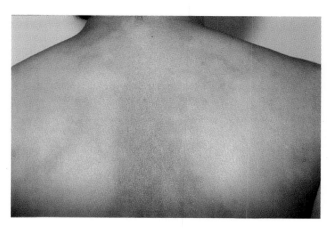

Plate 2 Hypopigmented macules of lepromatous leprosy in a Bangladeshi. The appearance is of BL, but histology showed downgrading to LL. Note the relative sparing of the midline.

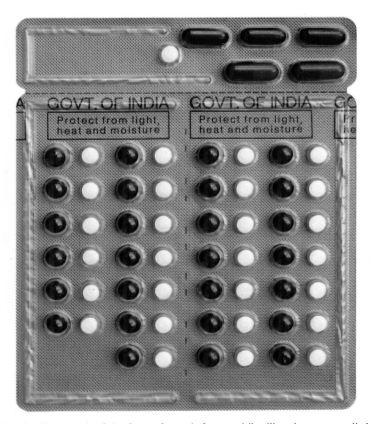

Plate 3 Photograph of the front of a pack form multibacillary leprosy supplied to the Government of India, showing the elevated 'blisters' or 'bubbles' that contain the supervised monthly dose (top right) and the tablets of dapsone and capsules of clofazimine for daily unsupervised dosage at home. The weeks are arranged in vertical columns and numbered on the reverse of the pack (see fig. 16.2 p. 221). Once the supervised drugs have been given, this part of the pack can be broken off along the horizontal line, and discarded. The rest of the pack is taken home by the patient. It may be folded along the central vertical line to fit into a coat or shirt pocket. Actual dimensions 122 × 146 mm. (Reproduced with kind permission from Georgiev & Kielstrup 1987 and with the cooperation of Pharmanova A/S, a division of Scanpharm)

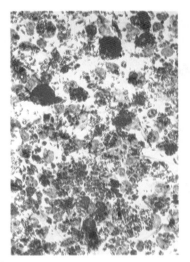

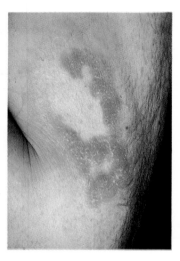

Plate 4 Acid-fast bacilli in the nose-blow smear from a patient with lepromatous leprosy.

Plate 5 Borderline tubercloid leprosy in reaction, in a European skin. Note the striking eruthema and slight scaling of the preexisting lesion, and the appearance of a new erythematous blush. The central area of healing remains inactive.

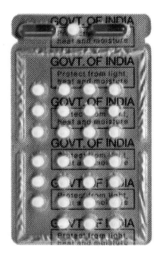

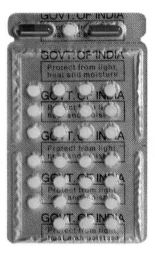

Plates 6 and 7 Packs for paubacillary leprosy: green for adults and blue for children. (Reproduced with the cooperation of Pharmanova A/S, a division of Scanpharm, Denmark).

1. Introduction

Definition

Leprosy is a chronic infectious disease of man caused by *Mycobacterium leprae*.

Leprosy is essentially a disease of peripheral nerves but it also affects the skin and sometimes certain other tissues, notably the eye, the mucosa of the upper respiratory tract, muscle, bone and testes.

History

There is a great deal of speculation about the early history of leprosy. The earliest records which give accurate descriptions of the disease come from India, and may have been written as early as 600 BC. Chinese records have also been found describing what appears to have been leprosy from a slightly later period. The descriptions of the disease which is called leprosy in the Bible do not correspond with the clinical picture of the disease, and probably encompass a varied group of skin conditions.

The earliest absolute evidence of leprosy is seen in an Egyptian skeleton of the 2nd century BC and in two Coptic mummies of the 5th century AD. It seems likely that leprosy reached the Mediterranean countries when the soldiers of Alexander the Great returned from India in 327–326 BC. It then spread slowly through the Greek and Roman Empires. The first known leprosy hospitals were established by Christians in Rome and Caesarea in the 4th century AD. The disease spread into Western Europe, reached epidemic proportions in the 12th–13th century, and then slowly declined. Leprosy evolves so slowly that its epidemiological pattern, which extended over several centuries, was much more poorly documented than that of acute diseases such as plague or typhus. In Norway the disease peaked in the 19th century, where Danielssen and Boeck wrote the first modern descriptions of the disease and Armauer Hansen carried out the first

1

bacterial and epidemiological research. Leprosy has died out completely in western and northern Europe over the last century, with the exception of Iceland, but it is still endemic at a low level in parts of southern and eastern Europe in small communities that have a low standard of living, poverty and crowded conditions, and in the Cajun community in Louisiana, USA.

At the present time leprosy is common in Asia, Africa and Central and South America. Its history in Africa is not known, but it was introduced into the Americas by Spanish and Portuguese settlers and their negro slaves, and by the French into Canada, where it has since died out. It is not known how leprosy reached the Australian aborigines. In this century small epidemics have occurred in several Pacific island communities where the disease was newly introduced.

From the earliest times leprosy has been a disease set apart from all others, and in a great many communities its sufferers and even those who cared for them have been rejected by society. For these and other reasons the enormous progress that has been made in medicine in this century has, until recently, passed leprosy by, and the few who devoted their lives to this disease have had to make do with inadequate staff, money, research and acknowledgement. Despite the fruitful yield of recent research, many enigmas remain and constitute a challenge to medicine.

Why was leprosy regarded as a special disease?

Some of the factors which have in the past set leprosy apart from other diseases are:

1. The extremely slow generation time of the bacillus. Most pathogens of man reproduce themselves in a matter of minutes, whereas *M. leprae* takes nearly two weeks. This results in a long incubation period, a very slow development of pathology, a slow and insidious clinical evolution and an unclear epidemiological pattern.

2. The bacillus has never been conclusively grown in artificial medium and consequently the bacteriology of leprosy was greatly delayed until 1960 when limited growth in mice was achieved.

3. This is the only bacillary disease with a predilection for nerve tissue. The factors determining this are unknown.

4. Man alone gets leprosy, and is the reservoir of infection, although naturally infected armadillos have been found in the southern USA, and primates in Africa.

5. Until very recently there was no satisfactory way of detecting

past or inapparent present infection. Epidemiological studies were therefore based largely on detection of clinical cases.

6. Leprosy is the best example of a disease which has a spectrum from complete absence of resistance by the host to effective immunity, which is often accompanied by extreme and destructive hypersensitivity. In lepromatous leprosy bacillary invasion is such that the number of bacilli in the dermis can reach 10^9 per gram of tissue. In tuberculoid leprosy on the other hand the cell mediated response to the presence of bacilli is so violent that it continues in the presence of a bacillary population which is too small to be detectable. The clinical patterns that result are so complex that until relatively recently they could not be understood.

7. Leprosy is unique in its psycho-social aspects. There is no other disease so associated with stigma and fear. This situation seems to be related to the fact that leprosy deforms and disables but seldom kills, so that those it has crippled live on, getting steadily worse, their deformities visible to all the community. Perhaps for this reason leprosy has commonly been considered to be a punishment from God. The attitude of society toward those suffering from leprosy has given rise to many unfortunate incidents of insult, rejection and even murder of patients, and in some societies these still continue. As for the patients themselves, they respond in various ways to the attitude society takes towards them. Some submit and accept while others take an attitude of anger and aggression toward mankind in general for the unjust persecution, or they take the role of the 'clown' to cope with the embarrassment caused by their unusual appearance. Occasionally they take their own lives as their only release from suffering.

The future

The objective appraisal and scientific investigation of leprosy, which began in 1873 with the discovery of the leprosy bacillus by Armauer Hansen in Norway, have received a great impetus in the past 30 years. The renaissance in immunology, cheap air fares, increasing student travel and the activities of the World Health Organization and other international and national agencies have all played their part. Scientific interest has increased knowledge and contributed to a reduction in stigma.

The discovery in 1941 of the value of sulphones in treating leprosy meant that for the first time thousands of patients could be successfully treated. This altered completely the pattern of care: leprosaria were closed, leprosy control became a realistic possibility and it began to dawn on patient and public alike that disability and deformity were not an inevitable sequel of the disease.

The introduction of multi-drug therapy in the 1980s prevented an epidemic of dapsone resistance and enhanced the quality and morale of control schemes. Animal models are providing essential clues about transmission. Sero-epidemiology opens up prospects for primary control, and molecular biology could lead to better diagnostic agents and vaccines.

There is no longer any need to regard leprosy as 'special'. The well-being of leprosy patients has become an integral part of the ordinary health service of many communities.

FURTHER READING

Andersen J G 1969 Studies in the mediaeval diagnosis of leprosy in Denmark. An osteoarchaeological, historical and clinical study. Danish Medical Bulletin 16 (suppl. 9): 1–142

Bechelli L M, Martinez Dominguez V 1966 The leprosy problem in the world. Bulletin of the World Health Organization 34: 811–826

Irgens L M 1973 Epidemiology of leprosy in Norway. International Journal of Epidemiology 2: 81–89

Møller-Christensen V 1953 Ten lepers from Naestved in Denmark. Danish Science Press, Copenhagen

Skinsness O K 1964 Leprosy in society. Leprosy Review 35: 21–35, 106–122, 175–181

World Health Organization Expert Committee on Leprosy, Sixth Report 1988 WHO Technical Report Series, 768. WHO, Geneva

2. *Mycobacterium leprae*

Classification

The genus *Mycobacterium* contain mycolic acid and sugars known as mycosides. Mycolic acid is responsible for the characteristic acid-fastness seen when the organism is stained with carbol-fuchsin. The genus is divided into two groups: fast growers that divide every few hours, and slow growers that divide about once a day. The fast growers are environmental bacteria, but some such as *M. chelionei* and *M. fortuitus* may cause skin sepsis or injection abscess in man. The slow growers are further grouped according to their production of pigment in culture. The non-chromögens include *M. ulcerans*, the cause of Buruli ulcer, and *M. tuberculosis*. *M. avium-intracellulare* (non-chromogen) and *M. kansasii* (photochromogen) may cause a disease resembling tuberculosis in man, especially in those with pre-existing lung disease or immune suppression. Other mycobacteria that cause disease in man are *M. marinum* (photochromogen) which is normally found in water and may cause a granulomatous skin lesion, and *M. scrofulaceum*, which is also found in soil and water and may cause lymphadenitis. Exposure to environmental mycobacteria may influence the response to subsequent exposure to *M. tuberculosis*, *M. leprae* and BCG (see Ch. 15).

M. leprae and *M. lepraemurium* (see 192) are classified separately because they have not yet been grown in culture.

Structure and composition

M. leprae is a straight rod about 1 to 8 μm long by 0.3 μm in diameter. In infected tissue the rods are often stacked or clumped together in globi. Electron-microscopy shows an ultrastructure common to all mycobacteria (Fig. 2.1).

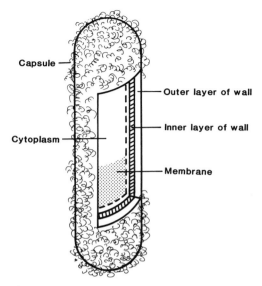

Fig. 2.1 Schematic structure of *Mycobacterium leprae.*

Capsule

Around the organism is an electron transparent zone of foamy or vesicular material, produced by and structurally unique to *M. leprae.* It is composed of two lipids, phthioceroldimycoserosate, which is thought to play a passive protective role, and a phenolic glycolipid, which is composed of three methylated sugar molecules linked through a phenol molecule to fat (phthiocerol). The trisaccharide renders it chemically unique and antigenically specific to *M. leprae* (Fig. 2.2).

Cell wall

This is composed of two layers:
   The outer layer is electron transparent and contains lipo-polysaccharide composed of branching chains of arabinogalactan esterified with long chain mycolic acids, similar to that found in other mycobacteria.
   The inner wall is composed of peptidoglycan: carbohydrate linked by peptides whose amino-acid sequence may be specific to *M. leprae* although the peptide is too scanty for use as a diagnostic antigen.

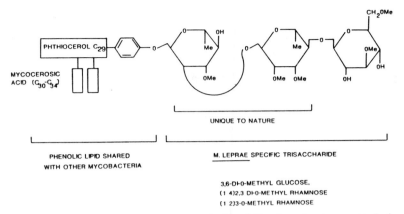

Fig. 2.2 Chemical structure of the trisaccharide of *Mycobacterium leprae*, attached to phenolic lipid (from Seckl, 1985)

Membrane

Just under the cell wall, and attached to it, is a membrane which is concerned with the transport of molecules into and out of the organism. The membrane is composed of lipid and proteins. The proteins are mostly enzymes and in theory constitute good targets for chemotherapy. They may also constitute the 'surface protein antigens' that have been extracted from the cell walls of disrupted *M. leprae* and extensively analysed (see p. 95).

Cytoplasm

The inner contents of the cell contain storage granules, deoxyribonucleic acid (DNA) the genetic material, and ribosomes which are proteins concerned with translation and multiplication. DNA analysis has been useful in confirming the identity as *M. leprae* of mycobacteria isolated from wild armadillos, and has shown that *M. leprae*, though genetically distinct, is closely related to *M. tuberculosis* and *M. scrofulaceum*.

Biochemistry and metabolism

Without access to cultured organisms this has been difficult to study. *M. leprae* metabolizes carbon sources through the classical pathways of glycolysis, the hexose monophosphate shunt and tricarboxylic acid cycles. Energy is stored by converting ADP to ATP, and produced by converting ATP to ADP. So oxygen is used. All bacteria need purine bases of nucleotides in order to make nucleic acids and for oxidative metabolism. Unlike other mycobacteria, *M. leprae* may not synthesize these and may have to scavenge them from the host cell. Mycobacteria also need iron which they extract and take up from the host by chelation with mycobactins. *M. leprae* lacks mycobactin. Metabolic defects such as these may perhaps explain why the organism has proved so difficult to culture in vitro.

Antigens

The main chemical constituents of *M. leprae* are antigenic (Table 2.1), but *M. leprae* contains relatively few antigens (about 20) that are recognized by antibodies in the serum of leprosy patients as compared with BCG (about 100), and many of them are weakly antigenic. Until 1981, when Brennan described the phenolic glycolipid and showed it was specific to *M. leprae*, all so-far identified antigens were widely cross-reactive with other mycobacteria, although some had a small part of the molecule, an epitope, that was specific to *M. leprae*. The epitope specificity enabled a specific antibody test to be established (see Ch. 7, p. 108) using sera that had been absorbed with other species of mycobacteria.

The antigenicity of *M. leprae* is dominated by the carbohydrate-containing antigens, which are physico-chemically stable.

Table 2.1 Antigens of *Mycobacterium leprae*. (This table does not provide a complete list of the antigens of *M. leprae*.)

Antigen	MW	Stability	Specificity	Immunoreactivity
Phenolic glycolipid I		Stable	*M. leprae*	IgM antibodies, suppressor T-cell responses
Other mycosides		Stable	Mycobacteria	?
Lipoarabinomannan	30–35 kd	Stable and indigestible	BCG and M.l. specific epitopes	IgG antibodies, T-cells, skin tests
Peptidoglycan		?	Mycobacteria	?
Proteins	65 kd 36 kd 28 kd 18 kd 12 kd	Labile	Common to other mycobacteria but have specific epitopes	Precipitating antibodies, T-cells, skin test (65 kd)

Phenolic glycolipid

The terminal trisaccharide confers antigenic specificity to *M. leprae*. Minor variants in the structure are designated I, II and III. The trisaccharide has been successfully synthesized and can be linked to a sample carrier protein for use in seroepidemiological and other studies, (see Ch. 15, p. 213). The antigen is found on all tissues infected with *M. leprae*, and persists there long after the organism has been killed. It is also found in the serum and urine of patients with lepromatous leprosy and its detection could become a useful diagnostic test for early lepromatous leprosy. The antigen stimulates IgM antibody production, but does not induce delayed hypersensitivity. It may play a role in inducing immune suppression in leprosy.

Lipoarabinomannan

This is the major component of the cell wall of *M. leprae*; it is stable and indigestible. It cross-reacts with other mycobacteria, but contains the specific epitopes recognized by absorbed sera, and induces IgG antibodies.

Protein antigens

There are many protein antigens in *M. leprae*, of which five have aroused particular interest because mouse monoclonal antibodies have shown that they contain *M. leprae* specific epitopes. Soluble proteins extracted from *M. leprae* have proved useful though not completely specific antigens for skin testing (see p. 113). Several protein antigens have been successfully cloned and expressed in *E. coli*, which greatly assists in their analysis.

Culture and identity

Attempts to culture *M. leprae* in vivo are considered in Chapter 14. In the absence of cultural characteristics, how may *M. leprae* be identified?

1. It is acid-fast when stained with carbol-fuchsin (see p. 60) and this acid-fastness may be removed or 'extracted' by pre-treatment with pyridine.
2. It will not multiply in conventional media that support the growth of other mycobacteria.
3. It will multiply in the footpads of mice, especially immuno-deficient mice, where it produces a characteristic histological pattern. Eventually it invades the peripheral nerves and causes leprosy (see p. 196).

4. It will multiply in armadillos, causing a characteristic disease (see p. 197).

5. It contains a unique glycolipid which can be identified serologically (see p. 108).

6. Its DNA may be extracted and shown to be homologous with that of established isolates of *M. leprae*.

Growth and death in vivo

In man, or other mammalian hosts, *M. leprae* is an obligate intracellular parasite. It multiplies mainly in histiocytes and Schwann cells, but may also do so in other cells including muscle cells and vascular endothelium (see p. 125) and, in the armadillo, in hepatocytes (see p. 197). Optimum temperature for growth is 30–33°C. Very little else is known of its growth requirements. In mice, and presumably in man, it divides every 12–13 days. No toxin has been identified, but its capsule may help protect it from chemical or immunological attack.

It is not known how *M. leprae* is killed. Most intracellular organisms are killed by H_2O_2 generated with macrophages that have been immunologically activated (see p. 103). But several species of mycobacteria are resistant to this mechanism. These mycobacteria may be digested by peroxidase in the presence of halide, but only young monocytes, not mature macrophages, can secrete this enzyme. In the absence of an effective immune response, as in lepromatous leprosy, most intracellular *M. leprae* probably live for about one year, and then start to degenerate. Staining with carbol-fuchsin shows irregular, then beaded, then granular organisms. Months or years after this stain fails to show them, skeletons of *M. leprae* may be seen in tissues by silver impregnation and the presence of their antigens demonstrated by immunofluorescence.

Susceptibility of *M. leprae* to physical and chemical agents outside the host is considered in Chapter 15.

FURTHER READING

Brennan P J 1986 Carbohydrate containing antigens of *Mycobacterium leprae*. Leprosy Review 57 (suppl. 2): 39–51

Draper P 1983 The bacteriology of *Mycobacterium leprae*. Leprosy Review 51: 563–575

Draper P 1986 Structure of *Mycobacterium leprae*. Leprosy Review 52 (suppl. 2): 15–20

Wheeler P R 1986 Enzymes and other biochemically active components of *Mycobacteria*. Leprosy Review, suppl. 2: 21–32

3. Clinical pathology

Most people who are infected with *M. leprae* develop a subclinical infection: that is to say they recover naturally without ever having symptoms or signs of disease. Few people develop the disease, leprosy. The clinical pattern of leprosy depends upon the response of the host to the organism.

M. leprae multiplies slowly, so leprosy develops slowly and its course is measured in months and years, as compared with hours and days in the case of acute bacterial disease.

Infection with *M. leprae* is usually considered to take place through the skin, or through the nasal mucosa from droplet infection (see Ch. 15). The earliest clinically detectable lesions are usually in the skin and, histologically, are in association with fine nerve fibres in the dermis which are most dense around the pilo-sebaceous follicles and their small blood vessels and with the erectores pilorum muscles. From the onset small cutaneous nerve fibres are involved. The organism multiplies best in the cooler parts of the body, so that the skin of the face and limbs and the more superficial nerves are preferentially invaded. Invasion of other organs takes place in lepromatous leprosy; the eye, testis and muscle being the most commonly affected. The bacillus multiplies inside macrophages, both those of the skin (histiocytes) and, especially, of the nerves (Schwann cells). As with other intramacrophage infections the effective host response is predominantly or even entirely cell mediated, as opposed to humoral. Compare the situation in leishmaniasis which is caused by an obligatory intracellular parasite in its vertebrate host, and in tuberculosis, brucellosis and typhoid which are caused by facultative intracellular organisms and have a similar host response.

Infecting organisms are taken up by histiocytes in the skin and, on penetrating terminal nerve twigs, by the Schwann cells. This usually elicits an inflammatory response of histiocytes and lymphocytes. Clinically there appears a small vague macule which is hypopigmented in a dark skin and erythematous in a light skin. The lesion is called

11

indeterminate as there is no indication how it will develop. Over 70% of indeterminate lesions in Africa heal spontaneously; many of them are never even noticed. If bacillary growth outstrips the defence mechanisms, whose nature in indeterminate leprosy is unknown, or if for some other reason the defence mechanisms fail, then the condition progresses into one of the patterns that make up the spectrum of disease in leprosy. The clinical pattern and ultimate outcome of the disease depend on the nature and extent of the host's response to the organism and upon the extent of bacilliary multiplication. The immune response of man to most, possibly all, bacterial infections is a dual one: humoral and cellular. The outcome of the disease in leprosy depends upon the degree to which cell mediated immunity develops or is suppressed (see Ch. 7). Antibody has not been shown to play any role in the defence against *M. leprae* but does contribute to the pathology and clinical picture of type 2 reactions (see Ch. 8).

(Some students may find it helpful to read the first part of Ch. 7 at this point).

Tuberculoid leprosy (TT)

When cell mediated immunity is well developed the pattern of disease is that of tuberculoid leprosy; the clinical picture reflects the tuberculoid histology. Macrophages take on the characteristics of epithelioid cells: nuclear chromatin becomes indistinct, cytoplasm becomes faintly acidophilic and granular and the cell membranes may fuse giving rise to Langhans' giant cells. Nests of epithelioid cells are surrounded by small lymphocytes. This arrangement is called a tubercle. In the skin, cellular infiltration may extend up to the epidermis and even involve the basal layer (Fig. 3.1). Cutaneous nerve twigs, both sensory and autonomic, are obliterated by the infiltrate, within and around the perineurium (Fig. 3.2), while larger nerves are swollen with oedema and epithelioid cells. Often only a few fascicles are infected, but inflammation in the epineurium and sheath causes compression within the sheath so that Schwann cells and axons are destroyed. Occasionally tubercles may caseate with the production of a sterile abscess within the nerve.

The disease is localized to one or a few sites in the skin and large peripheral nerves. Skin lesions are solitary and well defined. They tend to heal spontaneously from the centre. In severe cases the intense cellular infiltrate destroys the pilo-sebaceous follicles and sweat glands within the lesion.

Nerve lesions are also solitary, usually affecting either the cutaneous branches related to the skin patches or large mixed peripheral nerves. The nerves are greatly thickened because of the intense cellular infiltration, but are irregular or fusiform, and the pattern of involvement is not symmetrical. Nerve damage may be rapid, there is anaesthesia in the distribution of the nerve and, if the nerve involved has motor fibres, weakness and wasting of muscles. Autonomic damage is manifest by cyanosis and impaired sweating.

Over half of patients with tuberculoid leprosy have bacilli in striated muscle, which may be more numerous than in skin lesions. Acid-fast bacilli are only rarely detectable in the slit-skin smears from lesions of tuberculoid leprosy. The presence of cellular immunity is reflected in the positive lepromin test.

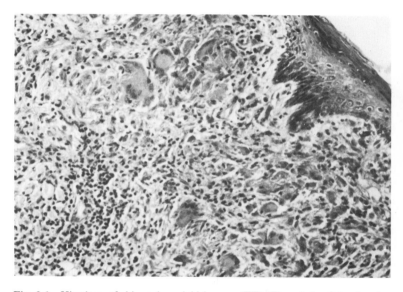

Fig. 3.1 Histology of skin, tuberculoid leprosy (TT). The whole of the dermis is infiltrated by the granuloma. There is no clear subepidermal zone. The granuloma consists of nests of epithelioid cells and lymphocytes. Many of the epithelioid cells have fused into Langhans' giant cells. They have pale bulky cytoplasm and relatively indistinct eccentric nuclei which in the giant cells are arranged in a half circle around the edge of the cells. Lymphocytes are clustered around the epithelioid cell nests. They are small with compact cytoplasm and dense dark staining nuclei. Nerve twigs are obliterated. A sweat gland, infiltrated with lymphocytes, can be seen bottom left. AFB could not be demonstrated by Ziehl-Neelsen's method. (Haematoxylin and eosin)

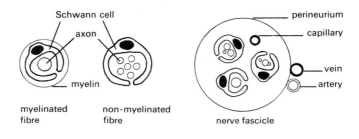

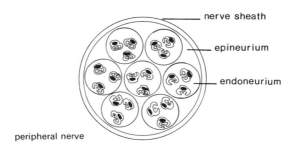

Fig. 3.2 The structure of a nerve, showing the relationship between axons, Schwann cells and perineurium.

Lepromatous leprosy (LL)

If cell mediated immunity fails to develop, the pattern of disease is that of lepromatous leprosy. The clinical picture reflects the enormous bacterial growth. The characteristic histological lesion is the leproma. In the skin, macrophages fail to specialize into epithelioid cells. Their shape varies from round to spindle, nuclear chromatin remains distinct and individual cells retain their identity. They become mere sacs to contain the multiplying bacilli; their cytoplasm undergoes fatty change and becomes oedematous, giving the appearance of the characteristic 'foam' cell. Bacilli may almost completely fill the cell, forming acid-fast globi (Fig. 3.3). Lymphocytes are absent or scanty and there is no attempt to surround macrophages. Dermal appendages are intact until late in the disease. The infiltrate does not, however, extend up to epidermis, but leaves a characteristic clear zone in which bacilli are only rarely seen (Fig. 3.4). Large numbers of bacilli are present in Schwann cells of cutaneous nerve fibres, in the surrounding endoneurial space, in myelinated axons, and in vascular endothelial cells. The perineurium leaks fluid, and a very few cells, usually macrophages, enter the nerve and take up bacilli. Later, perineurial

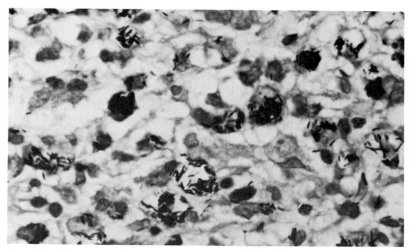

Fig. 3.3 Histology of skin, lepromatous leprosy (LL). High power view which shows the characteristic foam cells and globi. The infiltrate consists of macrophages with irregular nuclei and foamy cytoplasm, in many of which there are vacuoles. Acid-fast bacilli are seen as dark rods, either individually or in clumps as globi completely filling the cytoplasm. There are no lymphocytes. (Fite Faraco)

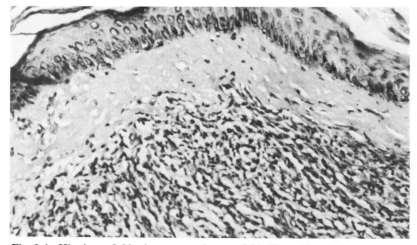

Fig. 3.4 Histology of skin, lepromatous leprosy (LL). The epidermis shows loss of rete ridges and is separated from the granuloma by a clear subepidermal zone, which characterizes lepromatous and borderline disease. There is a massive infiltrate of the dermis which consists of undifferentiated spindle-shaped macrophages, some of which are showing foamy degeneration of their cytoplasm. Ziehl-Neelsen's method revealed many acid-fast bacilli (BI 5+) but only a few small globi. This picture of very active disease is from a biopsy of a new nodule. in a patient relapsing while still on dapsone. (Haematoxylin and Eosin)

cells are invaded. In an infected nerve, all the fascicles are involved. (Fig. 3.5). Schwann cells reduplicate in an attempt to repair the damage and may form concentric rings around the nerve fibres, so creating an 'onion skin' appearance on histological sections. The influx of cells and fluid creates pressure inside the intact perineurium. Non-myelinated fibres are damaged more easily than myelinated fibres, but damage proceeds slowly and is followed, first by axonal degeneration and later, after several years, by hyaline degeneration and fibrosis of affected nerves. Bacilli multiply in Schwann cells, which then rupture. Phagocytosis of bacilli by other Schwann cells probably helps spread the infection centripetally along the nerves, but haematogenous spread is also important.

The disease is not localized and spreads rapidly, both locally and by the blood to other parts of the skin, to nerves, to the mucosa of the upper respiratory tract and to all the organs of the body, affecting particularly the eye, the testes, lymph nodes, the marrow of the phalanges and, to a lesser extent, superficially placed muscle, liver and spleen.

Clinically, the disease is characterized by multiplicity of lesions which are distributed all over the body in striking bilateral symmetry. The earliest lesions are small ill-defined macules which may be so

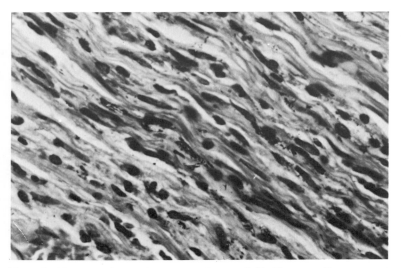

Fig. 3.5 Histology of nerve, lepromatous leprosy (LL). The nerve fibres are clearly seen and are partially separated by oedema. There is little or no lymphocytic infiltrate. Acid-fast bacilli are seen as dark rods, many of which are granular within the cytoplasm of Schwann cells, which are enlarged. At this stage nerve function is still almost normal. (Fite Faraco)

extensive that they coalesce (Plate 2). They are not anaesthetic because the nerves are not destroyed by cellular infiltration. As bacillary multiplication proceeds unhindered, the lesions become infiltrated and nodulation follows. Nasal mucosa is infiltrated early and is highly bacilliferous. Invasion of the larynx is a dangerous complication, which is seen more commonly in Asia than in Africa.

Involvement of nerves is likewise symmetrical. Nerve conduction studies show almost twice as many nerves are involved as can be detected by clinical examination. The most superficial fibres of cutaneous nerves in the coolest surfaces of the body are the first to become affected. Sensation is lost first to pin prick, temperature, and light touch and much later to deep pressure and other modalities. Gradual extension of nerve damage over many years finally results in total anaesthesia of limbs and even much of the trunk. When the appropriate level on large mixed peripheral nerves has been reached, motor damage will follow. Clinical tests show that autonomic nerves are damaged. Tendon reflex arcs are intact until very late in the disease.

Lepromatous leprosy is a systemic disease, with bacillaemia and multiple organ involvement.

The eye becomes infected both by local and haematogenous spread (see Ch. 11). Lepromata can form on the conjunctiva, and the cornea becomes hazy with keratitis. Corneal branches of the fifth nerve may be involved early. Bacilli invade the iris and form miliary lepromata round the pupil, and the ciliary body is slowly destroyed. Eye damage is remarkably insidious and slow, unless there is a reactional state which can produce acute iridocyclitis. Damage of the fifth and seventh nerves results in anaesthesia of the cornea and in lagophthalmos, predisposing the eye to trauma and infection, which may be worsened if the nasolacrimal duct is blocked by lepromatous granulation within the nose. Other cranial nerves are unaffected.

Both smooth and striated muscle are invaded, especially those lying superficially (Fig. 3.6). Arrectores pilorum and dartos muscles may contain many bacilli. Invasion of striated muscles of the face, hands and feet is a further cause of wasting and weakness and may be present before major nerve involvement. Bacilli seem to be protected in muscle, as they survive here long after they have been cleared by treatment from most other sites.

Veins in the limbs become tortuous with irregular lumen, narrowing and dilatation. Fibrosis and granulomas are seen, but bacilli are scanty, which suggests that the defects may be due to nerve damage.

Bones may be invaded in lepromatous leprosy. The nasal bones and

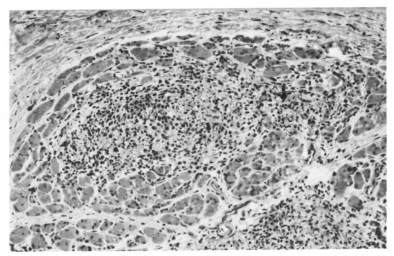

Fig. 3.6 Histology of hypothenar muscle, borderline lepromatous leprosy (BL). The bundles of muscle fibres are infiltrated with and separated by inflammatory cells, and are undergoing atrophy. The atrophy may be partly due to nerve damage. The infiltrate consists of histiocytes, plasma cells and lymphocytes. AFB can be demonstrated by Ziehl-Neelsen's method in some of the histiocytes and in a few muscle cells. The lymphocytic infiltrate is a borderline characteristic and the presence of necrosis and oedema suggest that the patient is having a reaction. (Haematoxylin and eosin)

the phalanges are those most commonly involved. Destruction of the anterior nasal spine leads to collapse of the nose, while destruction of the alveolar process of the maxilla allows the upper central incisor teeth to fall out (Fig. 3.7). The marrow of the phalanges is replaced with bacilli-laden foam cells which invade the cancellous bone and may form cysts within it and destroy it. Occasionally cortical bone is thinned. There is osteoporosis and the bone fractures easily. Fractures are often near joints, which collapse. The digits may become shortened and distorted. Joint cartilage may also be directly invaded, but only where the cartilage lies close under the surface of the skin. Likewise superficially placed tendons and tendon sheaths, such as those on the back of the wrist, may be infiltrated.

Nasal cartilage is commonly invaded and the septum may ulcerate, especially in the presence of secondary infection. The epiglottis is the commonest part of the larynx to be invaded.

The testis is the most commonly and severely affected viscus. The epithelial cells of the seminiferous tubules are invaded and aspermia and sterility ensue. Leydig cells undergo hypertrophy and eventual

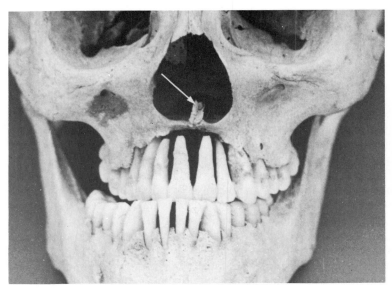

Fig. 3.7 Skull, lepromatous leprosy. The skull was one of a thousand dug up at the site of a medieval leprosarium, St Jørgen's Hospital, Naestved, Denmark. It shows one of the two characteristic changes: destruction of the alveolar process of the maxilla, exposing the roots of the upper central and lateral incisors which were held in place in this patient only by the soft tissues. The other structure frequently affected is the nasal spine (arrowed) which supports the tip of the nasal septum. (From the collection of Professor V. Møller-Christensen, Museum of Medical History, University of Copenhagen.)

destruction. The pathogenesis of gynaecomastia in lepromatous leprosy is presumed to be related to Leydig cell change. Liver damage and protein malnutrition may also contribute.

All lymph nodes draining the skin and many deeper nodes are invaded by macrophages, many of them containing acid-fast bacilli. The significance of this invasion is discussed in Chapter 7.

In the liver *M. leprae* are phagocytosed by and possibly multiply in Kupffer cells which may become the focus of multiple small granulomata. The kidney is not invaded by *M. leprae* but may be damaged by immune complex mediated glomerulonephritis (see p. 38).

Leprosy does not protect the patient against other diseases, and lepromatous disease may even lower resistance to infection (see p. 112).

Acid-fast bacilli are present in all lesions in lepromatous leprosy. Slit-skin smears are consistently positive, the Bacterial Index being 5 or 6 plus (see p. 63).

The absence of cellular immunity is reflected in the negative lepromin test. The immune response in lepromatous leprosy and the nature of the immunological defect are discussed in Chapter 7.

Amyloidosis

Secondary amyloidosis is one of the few fatal complications of leprosy (see p. 40). It occurs in patients with longstanding multi-bacillary disease, particularly those who suffer from recurrent type 2 reactions, and in any patient with chronic plantar ulcers. Insoluble amyloid fibrils are deposited in the major organs including kidneys, liver, spleen and adrenals causing irreversible dysfunction and failure. In secondary amyloidosis the amyloid fibrils are composed of amyloid A (AA) protein, as opposed to immunoglobulin light chains in primary (AL) amyloidosis. The precursor of AA protein is the acute phase serum protein SAA, whose concentration rises several hundredfold after injury or inflammation, including type 2 reactions. Those who develop secondary amyloidosis may have an enzyme defect such that they do not metabolize SAA completely, but produce the AA protein which polymerizes into insoluble fibrils. The diagnosis of amyloidosis is by histology of biopsies of rectum, kidney, subcutaneous fat or other affected tissues. When stained with Congo Red, and viewed under polarized light, amyloid tissue exhibits typical apple-green birefringence. In Papua New Guinea, 20% of patients with lepromatous leprosy for over two years had amyloidosis demonstrated by rectal biopsy.

Borderline leprosy (BB)

In between the two extreme, or polar, forms lies the rest of the spectrum of disease in leprosy, the clinical features of any particular point reflecting the balance between bacillary multiplication and cellular immunity in the individual patient (Fig. 3.9).

Histologically, macrophages have differentiated into epithelioid cells, but acid-fast bacilli are readily seen within them. Giant cells are unusual. Lymphocytes are usually present and loosely scattered throughout the epithelioid cell granuloma, but there is no focalization into tubercles. Nerves are infiltrated with mononuclear cells but are still recognizable. The clear subepidermal zone seen in lepromatous leprosy is still present.

The clinical features reflect the lack of focalization of the disease as

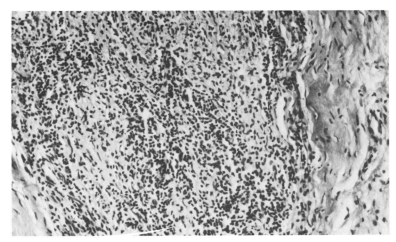

Fig. 3.8 Histology of nerve, borderline tuberculoid leprosy (BT). The contents of the nerve sheath are entirely replaced by a tuberculoid granuloma. Epithelioid cells are not as prominent as in Figure 3.1, but are still focalized by lymphocytes which compose the bulk of the lesion. (Haematoxylin and eosin)

well as the precarious nature of the balance. There are many skin lesions, of all shapes and sizes. Many nerves are involved, though not symmetrically as in lepromatous leprosy, nor does the patient have the complications associated with bacillary invasion.

Acid-fast bacilli are present, the Bacterial Index being 3 or 4 plus. The lepromin test is negative.

Most patients with leprosy show some borderline (or dimorphous as it is sometimes called) characteristics, and with clinical practice it is usually possible to say whether the patient lies near the middle of the spectrum (BB), towards the tuberculoid end (BT) or towards the lepromatous end (BL). Accurate determination of the exact position of the patient on the spectrum can be made histologically. Midpoint BB is almost a theoretical point on the spectrum. It is so unstable that the disease usually changes rapidly to BT or BL.

In *borderline tuberculoid* (BT) leprosy the granuloma is histologically like that seen in TT, but there is a clear narrow subepidermal zone. BT differs from BB in that the epithelioid cells are focalized by lymphocytes into tubercles, and Langhans' giant cells may be present. Nerves are moderately or severely infiltrated (Fig. 3.8). The Bacterial Index is not more than 1 or 2 plus and the lepromin test is weakly positive (1+ or 2+).

In *borderline lepromatous* (BL) leprosy the lesion contains more

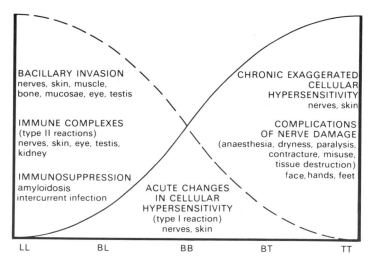

Fig. 3.9 Mechanisms of damage in leprosy, and tissues affected. Mechanisms under the broken line are characteristic of disease near the lepromatous end of the spectrum, those under the solid line of the tuberculoid end. They overlap in the centre where, in addition, instability predisposes to type 1 reactions.

lymphocytes than in LL, and there may be some early differentiation of macrophages towards epithelioid cells, but foamy change is common. The Bacterial Index is usually 4–5 plus and the lepromin test is negative.

Mechanisms by which tissues are damaged in leprosy are summarized in Figure 3.9.

VALUE OF CLASSIFICATION

It is useful to be able to assess accurately the patient's position on the spectrum, to classify his disease, for several reasons.

1. An understanding of the spectral concept must precede an awareness of the multiplicity of the clinical manifestations of the disease, if the diagnosis of leprosy is to be correctly made.

2. Tuberculoid (TT and especially BT) leprosy is associated with severe large nerve damage: lepromatous leprosy, with chronicity and long-term complications.

3. Near the tuberculoid pole healing usually occurs spontaneously; this rarely happens near the lepromatous pole.

4. Polar forms of the disease tend to be immunologically 'stable'

and are unlikely to change their position on the spectrum, which means that type 1 reactional states (see Ch. 8) are not encountered.

5. Borderline disease is unstable and may move either way along the spectrum. Such a shift in cellular immunity is often accompanied by an acute reaction (type 1). These reactions, which may occur spontaneously or be precipitated by treatment, are likely to be associated with severe multiple nerve damage.

6. Lepromatous patients are likely to suffer reactions mediated by antigen-antibody complexes (type 2).

Correct positioning of the patient's disease on the spectrum at diagnosis will therefore help in determining the likely response to and duration of treatment, and the complications likely to be encountered so that proper precautions can be taken to prevent them. Additionally,

7. For research purposes classification provides a basis for matching patients in studies such as drug trials.

8. Classification of patients seen during a leprosy survey may help in planning control measures.

FURTHER READING

Bernard J C, Vasquez C A J 1973 Visceral lesions in lepromatous leprosy. International Journal of Leprosy 41: 94–101

Dastur D K, Ramamohan Y, Dabholkar A S 1974 Some neuropathologic and cellular aspects of leprosy. Progress Research 18: 53–75

Date A, Harrihar S, Jeyvarthini S E 1985 Renal lesions and other major findings in necropsies of 133 patients with leprosy. International Journal of Leprosy 53: 455–460

Desikan K V, Job C K 1968 A review of postmortem findings in 37 cases of leprosy. International Journal of Leprosy 36: 32–44

Holla V V, Kenetkar M V, Kholhatkar M K, Kulkarin C N 1983 Leprous synovitis. A study of fifty cases. International Journal of Leprosy 51: 29–32

Job C K, Karat A B A, Karat S, Mathan M 1969 Leprosy myositis — a histopathologic and electron microscopic study. Leprosy Review 40: 9–16

Johny K V, Karat A B A, Rao P S S, Date A 1975 Glomerulonephritis in leprosy — a percutaneous renal biopsy study. Leprosy Review 46: 29–37

McAdam K P W J, Anders R F, Smith S R, Russell D A, Price M A 1975 Association of amyloidosis with erythema nodosum reactions and recurrent neutrophil leucocytosis. Lancet 2: 572–575

Mitsuda K, Ogawa M 1937 A study of one hundred and fifty autopsies on cases of leprosy. International Journal of Leprosy 5: 53–60.

Møller-Christensen 1961 Bone Changes in Leprosy. John Wright, Bristol

Pearson J H M, Weddell A G M 1975 Perineurial changes in untreated leprosy. Leprosy Review 46: 51–67

Pearson J M H, Rees J J W, Weddell A G M 1970 Mycobacterium leprae in striated muscle of patients with leprosy. Leprosy Review 41: 155–167

Pedley J C, Harman D J, Waudby H, McDougall A C 1980 Leprosy in peripheral nerves: histopathological findings in 119 untreated patients in Nepal. Journal of Neurology, Neurosurgery and Psychiatry 43: 198–204

Ridley D S 1974 Histological classification and the immunological spectrum of leprosy. Bulletin of the World Health Organization, 51: 451–465

Ridley D S, Jopling W H 1966 Classification of Leprosy according to immunity, a five-group system. International Journal of Leprosy 34: 255–273

Shepard C C 1965 Temperature optimum of *M. leprae* in mice. Journal of Bacteriology 90: 1271–1275

4. Symptoms and signs

The clinical features of leprosy reflect the pathology, which is in turn dependent upon the balance between bacillary multiplication and the host's cell mediated immune response.

INCUBATION PERIOD

The slowness of onset, insignificance of early clinical signs and difficulty of experimental transmission in man make it impossible to assess the incubation period accurately, either in a population or in an individual.

Two to four years is considered usual, although periods from three months to 40 years have been recorded.

PRESENTATION

Skin lesions

There may be a single patch or several lesions. Some patients give a history of one lesion being present for several years before the appearance of others, or of the initial lesion having disappeared spontaneously some months or years before the subsequent lesions appeared. In others the disease spreads immediately from the primary lesion. Some patients do not notice their lesions until they become inflamed during a reaction.

Classically the first lesion is of *indeterminate leprosy* (Fig. 4.1). It appears as a symptomless ill-defined slightly hypopigmented macule a few centimetres across. It is commonly seen on the face, trunk or extensor surfaces of the limbs. Sometimes there are several lesions. Sensation is normal or only slightly impaired; sweating and hair growth are usually unaffected. Bacilli are difficult to find and diagnosis may depend on careful continuing observation. Many patients, however, do not present until lesions have developed characteristics determinate of some point on the spectrum.

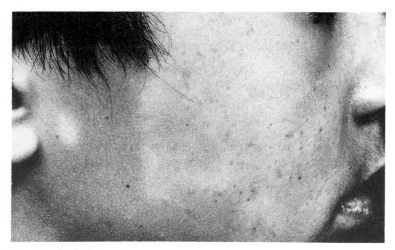

Fig. 4.1 An indistinct hypopigmented macule, with a satellite in front of the ear, was the only sign of leprosy in this Nepali child.

Numbness

Anaesthesia is common but it is surprising how seldom anaesthesia brings the patient to the doctor. More commonly the patient cuts or burns his hand or foot without noticing it at the time and he may not realize that the limb is anaesthetic until asked if the injury hurt him. Numbness of an individual skin lesion is a common presentation, especially in Asia.

Weakness

Muscular weakness may be slow in onset or sudden. In borderline and tuberculoid leprosy, damage to a large peripheral nerve may be gradual and weakness may occasionally be present before anaesthesia is noticed. More commonly an acute reaction may precipitate a sudden motor paresis causing, in particular, ulnar palsy, foot drop or facial palsy and this may be the first indication. In lepromatous leprosy bacillary invasion of muscle may cause weakness of face, feet or hands.

Pain

Pain in one or several nerves may be the presenting symptom in tuberculoid or borderline tuberculoid leprosy even before skin lesions have appeared. Painful lymphadenopathy secondary to infection in an anaesthetic limb may call attention to its cause in a wound of hand or foot.

Eyes

Pain, photophobia and blurred vision may be the first indication of iridocyclitis in lepromatous leprosy (see Ch. 11).

Nose

Nasal stuffiness, discharge, or bleeding may be the first symptom of lepromatous leprosy.

Systemic symptoms

Occasionally, fever, malaise, joint pains, arthritis, tenosynovitis, myositis or lymphadenitis accompanying a reaction is the first manifestation of leprosy.

Itching

Rarely, a short period of generalized itching may herald the onset of diffuse rapidly progressive lepromatous leprosy, before skin changes are visible.

EVOLUTION OF DISEASE

Entry into the spectrum

Perhaps three out of four indeterminate lesions heal spontaneously. The rest become determinate and enter the clinical spectrum. Increasing definition, hypopigmentation, hyperaesthesia, anaesthesia or elevation of margin indicate movement towards the tuberculoid pole, while increase in numbers of lesions, erythema and vagueness or central elevation indicate movement towards the lepromatous pole (see Table 4.1). As the disease progresses, or reactions develop (se p. 115), macular lesions may give way to infiltrated lesions (Fig. 4.2).

Characteristics of disease at different points along the spectrum

The definition of points on the spectrum is to some extent arbitrary, with the exception of the lepromatous pole where there is a complete

Table 4.1   Clinical characteristics of leprosy at the poles

	Lepromatous	Tuberculoid
Skin and nerves		
Number and distribution	Widely disseminated	One or a few sites, asymmetrical
Skin lesions		
Definition:		
Clarity of margin	Poor	Good
Elevation of margin	Never	Common
Colour: dark skin	Slight hypopigmentation	Marked hypopigmentation
light skin	Slight erythema	Coppery or red
Surface	Smooth, shiny	Dry, scaly
Central healing	None	Common
Sweat and hair growth	Impaired late	Impaired early
Loss of sensation	Late	Early and marked
Nerve enlargement and damage	Late	Early and marked
Bacilli (Bacterial Index)	Many (5 or 6+)	Absent (0)
Natural outcome	Progression	Healing

absence of cell mediated immunity, and which is fixed. The clinical spectrum, although linear, overlies a number of 'bulges'; 'bulges' of bacillary invasion, of cellular immunity, of instability, of liability to nerve damage, and of liability to a rapid downhill course. The bulges, and the characteristics of the disease overlying them, need to be identified.

It is important to distinguish in one's mind between the identification of the position of a patient's disease on the LL–TT spectrum, a process which in addition to full clinical examination may require bacteriology, skin testing and histology, and the simple description of a *skin lesion* which may be tuberculoid, borderline or lepromatous in appearance. An appreciation of this point makes it possible to accommodate without confusion much of the older terminology, which was based mainly on clinical observations. One valuable aspect of older terminologies, some of which are mentioned below in parentheses, was that they enabled a particular set of signs to be recognized as indicating a particular natural outcome of the disease.

Tuberculoid leprosy (TT)

Skin lesions are few in number. Often there is only one. They are

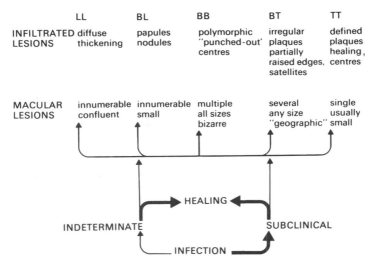

Fig. 4.2 Movement into spectrum and main features of skin lesions. At the lepromatous end there is usually a progression from macules to nodules; at the tuberculoid end plaques may arise independently of macules.

seldom over 10 cm in diameter. They are not symmetrical on the body and may cross the midline. They are hypopigmented in dark skins, sometimes copper coloured in pale skins, and easy to see (Plate 1). The margin is well defined and unbroken. They may be macular or raised, either as a plaque or at the edge, where the disease is progressing while the centre is flat indicating healing (Figs. 4.3–4). The lesions are anaesthetic, hairless and dry as sweating is impaired. Lesions on the face are not as likely to be as insensitive as those elsewhere because of the rich overlapping nerve supply to the skin of the face.

Tuberculoid skin lesions which are small, markedly hypopigmented and pebbled and which proceed to rapid central healing (minor tuberculoid) are not usually associated with severe nerve involvement (Fig. 4.3). Large lesions, which tend to be more numerous and are more markedly and uniformly raised (major tuberculoid) are more often associated with severe nerve involvement. These latter lesions may also invade the 'spared areas' (see p. 34), especially the scalp, axillae, groins, palms and soles (Fig. 4.5). The clinical descriptive terms major and minor tuberculoid refer to lesions in BT patients.

Solitary peripheral nerves are commonly enlarged in tuberculoid leprosy and may, on occasion, be the only sign of disease (Fig. 4.6). Sites of predilection are, in order of frequency: the ulnar nerve immediately

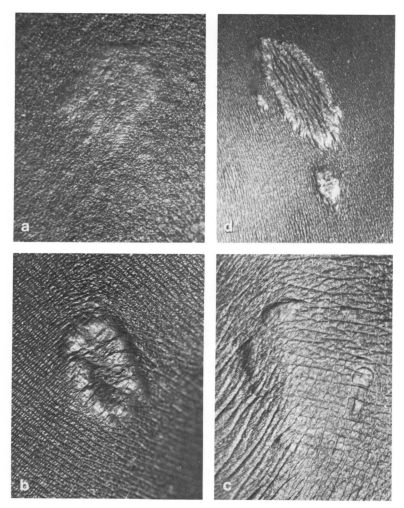

Fig. 4.3   Four typical lesions of tuberculoid leprosy.
a   This solitary hypopigmented plaque on the cheek of a girl was anaesthetic.
Note the clear markings and definition. There were no other signs of leprosy
(TT);
b   This young woman had 3 such anaesthetic skin lesions, with raised succulent
edges and depressed centres suggesting early healing (TT);
c   The lesion here has almost healed, leaving only a thin raised edge round
apparently normal skin. But sensation was impaired and the radial cutaneous
nerve was enlarged (TT);
d   This plaque is also well defined, and its edge is raised and scaly. The centre
is rough, dry and anaesthetic. Two small satellite lesions indicate local spread of
the disease; this is a borderline characteristic and suggests BT rather than TT. A
biopsy would be necessary for precise classification.

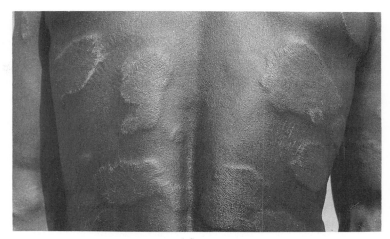

Fig. 4.4 Borderline tuberculoid leprosy (BT). These lesions show many TT features but they are numerous, large and irregular, characteristics which imply that the patient's defences are not controlling the disease. Despite the extensive skin disease, nerve damage was slight.

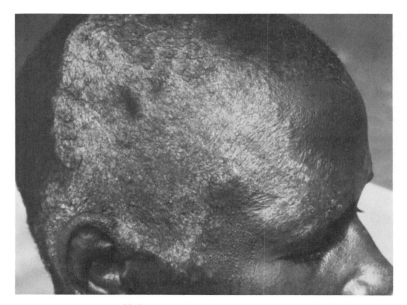

Fig. 4.5 Major tuberculoid leprosy (BT). This large lesion on the scalp is typical of major tuberculoid leprosy. The edge is raised, pebbled and well defined. The surface is scaly, even crusty behind the ear, indicating that there has been a reaction to which this type of lesion is particularly prone. Several peripheral nerves were greatly enlarged and tender.

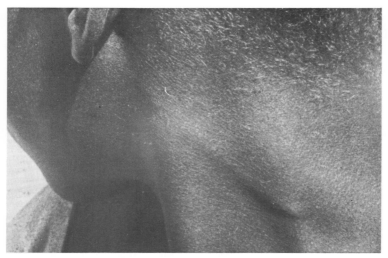

Fig. 4.6   Borderline tuberculoid leprosy (BT). The great auricular nerve is visible as it runs upwards and forwards across the sterno-mastoid muscle. This nerve may be palpable in a thin person.
Enlargement of this nerve often, but not always, accompanies a cutaneous lesion on the side of the face. The nerve has no motor fibres and its involvement is unimportant except as a diagnostic pointer.

above the olecranon groove, the posterior tibial nerve behind the internal malleolus, the common peroneal (lateral popliteal) nerve in the popliteal fossa and proximal to where it winds round the neck of the fibula, the radial cutaneous nerve at the wrist, the facial and great auricular nerves, and the median nerve proximal to the flexor retinaculum. In addition any cutaneous branch associated with a patch may be enlarged. Nerve enlargement usually precedes the signs of nerve damage in tuberculoid leprosy unless the disease presents in an acute reaction when enlargement, tenderness, pain and paresis all appear suddenly together. With early diagnosis and proper treatment nerve damage can be avoided. Consequently, signs of nerve damage are considered as complications (see Ch. 10).

Tuberculoid leprosy (TT) represents the top of the bulge of cellular immunity (Fig. 4.7), the features of which are stability of disease, absence of dissemination or of local spread, infrequency of reactions and tendency to spontaneous healing. Treatment is usually given however in order to minimize nerve damage. Tuberculoid leprosy presenting with macular lesions (maculoanaesthetic) can heal spontaneously without the lesions ever becoming infiltrated.

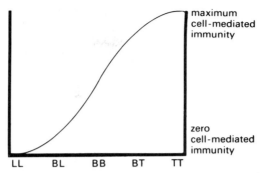

Fig. 4.7 The bulge of cell mediated immunity. Note the steepness of the slope in the middle of the spectrum.

Lepromatous leprosy (LL)

Lepromatous leprosy represents the top of the bulge of bacillary multiplication (Fig. 4.8), which accounts for many of the features of the disease at this pole and for many of the complications: insidious onset, steady downhill course, multiple organ involvement, facial deformity and blindness. Lepromatous leprosy also predisposes the patient to the complications of antigen-antibody reactions and immune complex disease.

The early lesions of lepromatous leprosy are macules (Fig. 4.9, Plate 2). They are widely disseminated, bilaterally symmetrical and innumerable. The edges are indistinct, and their surface shiny and erythematous rather than hypopigmented. In rapidly progressive cases

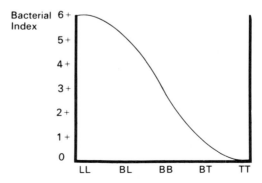

Fig. 4.8 The bulge of bacillary multiplication. Note how steeply the Bacterial Index rises between BT and BL.

they coalesce so that the whole skin is uniformly affected, and even in a good light the lesions are difficult to see. Certain areas of skin, notably the scalp, axillae and groins, palms and soles, antecubital and popliteal fossae and midline of the back are spared until late in the disease. These areas of skin are the warmest. The early macules of lepromatous leprosy are not anaesthetic.

The manifestations of nerve damage are relatively slow to appear. Sensory loss is symmetrical and is first detected over the extensor surfaces of the forearm, leg, hand and foot. These areas grow slowly in size to cover the rest of the arms, legs and buttocks and then spread onto the trunk, but sparing the areas mentioned above, which do not become anaesthetic unless and until the large peripheral nerves are involved. This is therefore not in its early stages a true glove and stocking distribution as in other forms of peripheral neuritis, and pain is unusual. Weakness usually starts in the intrinsic muscle of hands and feet.

If the disease is allowed to progress untreated, the affected skin takes on a waxy appearance and feels full. Thickening is most marked over the face, especially the forehead, earlobes, eyebrows, nose and malar

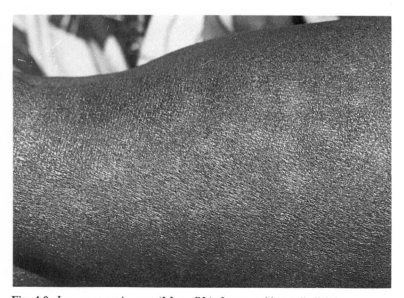

Fig. 4.9 Lepromatous leprosy (LL or BL). Innumerable small slightly hypopigmented macules cover the upper arm. Similar macules were seen on the trunk, buttocks, thighs and face. The lesions were not anaesthetic but skin smears had a bacterial index of 5+.

surfaces (Figs. 4.10, 4.11). The thickened skin starts to develop into folds, which hang down producing the classical lion-like, or leonine, facies. The eyebrows and eyelashes are lost, a condition known as madarosis. Nodulation of these areas may follow and similar changes develop over other areas of affected skin. Nodules are raised centrally and slope off gradually. By this time anaesthesia is extensive and is accompanied by anhydrosis. Excessive compensatory sweating from unaffected areas, especially the axillae, becomes obvious, and probably underlies the popular belief in some countries that sweating is a sign of leprosy.

Lymph nodes are palpable enlarged in 90% of patients with LL, as compared with about 70% in paucibacillary disease. The order of frequency is inguinal, cervical, axillary, epitrochlear.

Invasion of the mucosa of the nose, and sometimes throat, accompanies invasion of the skin in about 80% of lepromatous patients and once started can progress rapidly. Nasal stuffiness, as with a common cold, may be the first symptom, and the mucosa looks thickened and pale yellow. Nodules or plaques form, which later obstruct the nose (Fig. 4.12). Minor trauma and secondary infection cause ulceration, epistaxis, muco-purulent discharge and the formation

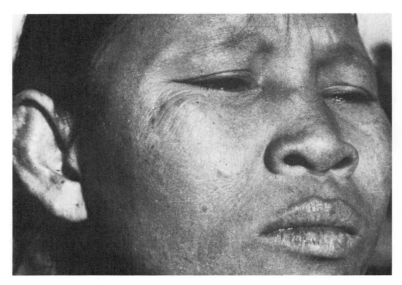

Fig. 4.10   Lepromatous leprosy (LL). There is diffuse infiltration of the face giving a plump waxy appearance to the cheeks, and loss of eyebrows. Note the nodule on the pinna. Smears were everywhere positive (BI 6+).

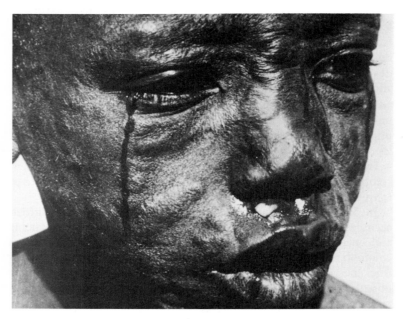

Fig. 4.11 Lepromatous leprosy (BL/LL). The infiltration has progressed much further than in the patient in Figure 4.10. Lacrimation is the consequence of iridocyclitis. The nasal discharge was teeming with *M. leprae*, making this patient highly infectious.

of crusts. Septal perforation follows unless the condition is treated vigorously. In late cases the anterior nasal spine is destroyed and the nose collapses. By this time there may be infiltration of the palate and larynx, with hoarseness and the danger of laryngeal obstruction. Rarely the palate may perforate.

Eye damage is considered in Chapter 11.

In advanced lepromatous leprosy the hands and feet become swollen, tense and oedematous. Radiography of the hands and feet shows osteoporosis of the phalanges with loss of trabeculation (the so-called 'ground glass' appearance) and often hairline fractures to which these bones are prone (Fig. 4.13). Nutrient foramina are enlarged. More rarely there are small osteolytic lesions, which may also predispose to compression fractures and swelling of the joints. These changes can produce shortening of the digits, a process which may be accelerated by the even more damaging mechanisms of pressure necrosis, trauma and infection, complications which are liable to follow anaesthesia in a patient who does not know how or neglects to take care of his

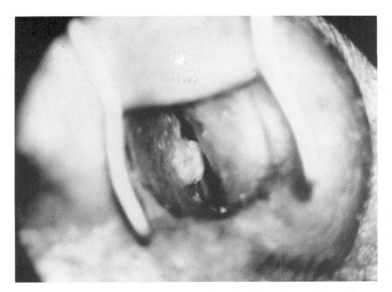

Fig. 4.12 Nose, lepromatous leprosy. Examination through a nasal speculum shows a pale nodule on the nasal septum. The mucosa is infiltrated and superficially ulcerated. Aerosols created by sneezing will contain millions of *M. leprae*.

anaesthetic limbs (see Ch. 10). Nail growth may be affected, the nails becoming curved, brittle and thin. Autonomic nerve damage may affect the cardiovascular response to posture and exercise.

Testicular damage is insidious and without symptoms unless the testes become acutely inflamed during a reaction. They are soft and small on palpation. Gynaecomastia may follow testicular atrophy, and is found in about one-third of men with longstanding LL, especially those who have experienced type 2 reactions (see p. 121). This dual condition is associated with increased excretion of urinary gonadotrophins and low plasma testosterone and urinary 17-ketosteroid levels, a condition likened to Kleinfelter's syndrome. Azoospermia and sterility usually precede the hormonal changes, which, in addition to causing gynaecomastia, may contribute to osteoporosis and possibly impotence.

Lepromatous leprosy is a 'stable' disease in that natural remission does not take place. Before the days of effective treatment bacillary multiplication continued inexorably. The downhill course was punctuated by bouts of acute inflammation at the sites of disease accompanied by crops of painful red lumps in the skin and systemic illness with fever (type 2 reactions: see p. 121). The commonest causes

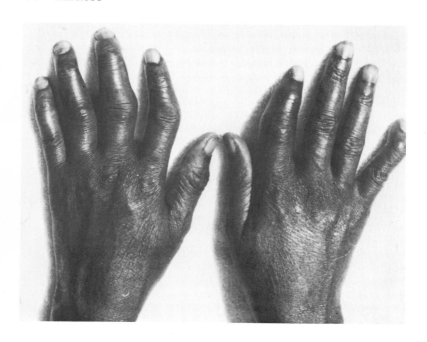

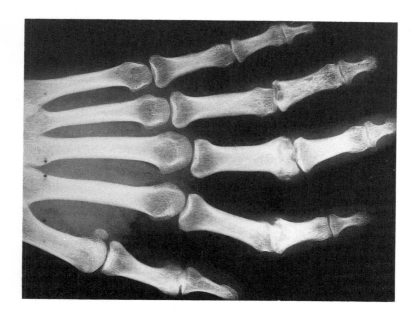

of death from leprosy are renal failure (10–40%: glomerulonephritis, interstitial nephritis, amyloidosis in one-third), acute infections (15–25%: especially pneumonia and tetanus and septicaemia following pyogenic infections of wounds in anaesthetic limbs), tuberculosis (10–30%: this figure was much higher before the days of anti-tuberculous chemotherapy), and the complications of old age (see Table 4.2). Nephritis and pneumonia are especially associated with lepromatous leprosy. Amyloid deposits are often widespread in lepromatous patients. Death from respiratory obstruction, hyper-pyrexia and cachexia are seldom seen any longer. These fatal complications can be prevented by early diagnosis and proper treatment.

Lucio leprosy. This is the purest form of lepromatous LL, and causes a slowly progressive diffuse shiny infiltration of the skin of the face and most of the body: (lepra bonita beautiful leprosy). Eyelids thicken and eyebrows fall out (sleepy or sad leprosy). Nasal congestion, hoarse voice, numbness and oedema of hands and feet eventually

Table 4.2 Complications of leprosy, from the post-mortem studies of Hansen & Looft (1895)

	Lepromatous (Nodular) 89 cases	Tuberculoid (Maculo-anaesthetic) 36 cases
Pneumonia	25%	8%
Tuberculosis	46%	42%
Nephritis	20%	8%
Fatty degeneration of kidneys	18%	28%
Amyloidosis	55%	28%
Others	7%	29%

Figures indicate the percentage of patients in whom the given pathology was found at autopsy. Most patients had more than one complication. The immediate cause of death was not specified. Note the increased prevalence of nephritis, pneumonia and amyloidosis in (untreated) lepromatous patients.

Fig. 4.13 Lepromatous leprosy (opposite). The hands are swollen and the fingers spindle shaped. Hypothenar muscles are wasted. The radiograph of the left hand shows how the deformities have developed. There is decalcification of the ends of the bones and reduced medullary trabeculation in the metacarpals, contrasting with increased cortical density of the shafts of some of the phalanges. These two signs indicate disuse and misuse respectively. There are cysts in several phalanges close to the proximal interphalangeal joints, due to leprous infiltration. Anaesthesia has permitted minor trauma to fracture the weakened bone close to these joints, causing angulation and shortening of the fingers. These changes have taken place without ulceration or secondary infection.

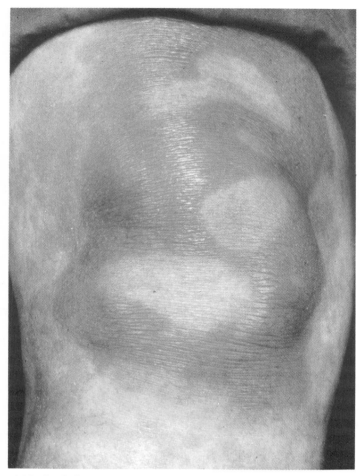

Fig. 4.14 Borderline leprosy (BB). The knee of this Saudi-Arabian woman shows a classical lesion. In the centre of a succulent red plaque are well-defined 'punched out' areas of apparently normal skin. The outer margin of the lesion is indistinct, fading gradually into normal skin which contains numerous erythematous macules, papules and plaques.

develop, but may be confused with myxoedema. This form of LL is liable to the most severe of all reactional states, the Lucio phenomenon (see Ch. 8). Lucio leprosy occurs in Mexicans of mixed Spanish and Amerindian ancestry, but is rare elsewhere.

Borderline leprosy (BB)

The clinical features of the centre of the spectrum show a mixture of the characteristics of disease at the poles, and are often bizarre and confusing.

There are many skin lesions, though not as numerous as in LL. There is a tendency to symmetry; some lesions may cross the midline. Macules vary greatly in size and shape, some may be well-defined, others poorly, others will have long streaming extensions like coastal inlets and headlands on a map. Satellites, like off-shore islands, are common. Raised lesions have the succulence, shine and sloping external edges of lepromatous lesions, but centrally there is often dimpling, a deeply punched-out area or frank healing as in a tuberculoid lesion (Fig 4.14). The presence of such a markedly tuberculoid characteristic suggests that the disease may have begun nearer that pole and subsequently 'downgraded' across the centre of the spectrum. Skin lesions are hypaesthetic.

Many nerves are affected, in an asymmetrical pattern. Enlargement may be smooth and regular, or lumpy and irregular. Anaesthesia, in the distribution of the nerves, appears early.

Signs suggesting bacillary invasion of nasal mucosa, eyes, bones and testes are usually absent.

Borderline leprosy represents the instability peak (Fig. 4.15). The balance between bacillary multiplication and cellular immunity is a delicate and precarious one and seldom lasts long without one or other feature gaining the upper hand. The character of the patient's disease then alters accordingly and a mixture of old and new features is seen.

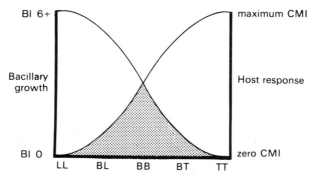

Fig. 4.15 The instability peak in borderline leprosy. Disease within the shaded area, where neither bacillary growth nor cell mediated immunity has the upper hand, is unstable: the steeper the slope the greater the instability.

Sometimes the picture is complex and histological examination may be necessary to identify the new position on the spectrum. This change may take place quietly, but often it takes place rapidly and is accompanied by inflammation within the lesions, a manifestation of acute cellular hypersensitivity (type 1 reaction: see p. 116).

This tendency to reaction, which is accompanied by rapid damage to nerves and skin, is the important characteristic of BB leprosy.

Instability at the centre of the spectrum may also account for another feature of leprosy: that although borderline disease (BL or BT) is always more common than polar disease, true BB without a preponderance of either L or T features is relatively rare. The distribution patterns for Asia, where lepromatous disease is relatively more common, and for Africa, where tuberculoid disease is relatively more common, are approximately represented in Fig. 4.16.

Approximate proportion of patients

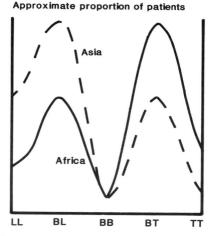

Fig. 4.16 Effect of the instability peak on patterns of leprosy in South-east Asia and in Africa.

Borderline tuberculoid leprosy (BT)

The features here are a mixture of those attributable to intense cellular infiltration and to those of the unstable centre.

The skin lesions resemble those of tuberculoid leprosy, but there is always evidence that the disease is not being contained. This may be apparent in either of two ways: individual skin lesions do not show the absolute *marginal definition* that characterizes TT. The edge may in part grade imperceptibly into normal skin, it may stream, or there may be small satellite lesions (Figs. 4.17, 4.18, 4.19). Elevated margins fall away in places like erosions in the rim of an old volcanic crater. Alternatively the lesions are *too numerous* for TT, and may show variation in size, contour and character (Figs. 4.4, 4.20). Such lesions are presumed to indicate a phase of haematogenous spread. Often both characteristics of BT are present. Skin lesions, except for some on the face, are insensitive, though less intensely so than in TT. Hypopigmentation, dryness, pebbling and scaling are less conspicuous than in TT (Fig. 4.21). In pale skins lesions are often red or copper coloured (Plates 1, 5).

Nerve lesions are more numerous than in TT. Several of the large peripheral nerves are likely to be irregularly enlarged at the sites of predilection and in an asymmetrical pattern. In long-standing cases almost all the peripheral nerves may be involved. Nerve damage is the most important characteristic of BT leprosy and anaesthesia or paresis in the distribution of a nerve is often found when the patient first presents. Patients may show evidence of typical nerve damage in the absence of skin lesions, and be difficult to diagnose.

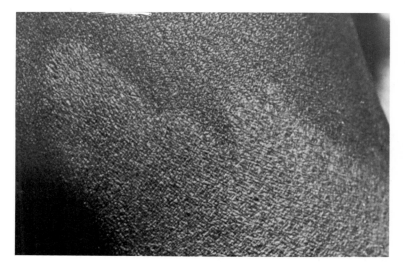

Fig. 4.17   Borderline tuberculoid leprosy (BT). This is the edge of a large macule which covers the posterior aspect of the upper arm of a 12-year-old child. The pale, rough surface, which was anaesthetic, is dry and hairless. The edge, though well defined for the most part, is streaming in places, showing that the infection is not being efficiently localized (BI 1+).

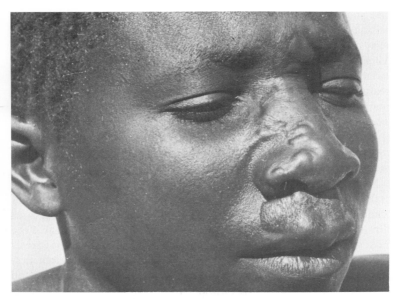

Fig. 4.18 Borderline tuberculoid leprosy (BT). This lesion is in the middle of the face, raised and generally well defined — tuberculoid characteristics; but is also oedematous due to type 1 reaction, the degree of elevation varies and the edge is irregular and in places unclear, fading imperceptibly into normal skin — borderline characteristics. The lesion was anaesthetic and AFB were present (BI 3+) indicating downgrading. Several nerves were involved.

Pure neural leprosy. Occasionally patients show evidence of typical nerve damage without skin lesions. This presentation is said to be more common in India than elsewhere. Usually only one nerve is involved, typically the ulnar at the elbow. Accurate diagnosis is essential to avoid disastrous mismanagement. Biopsy may be necessary, and histology most commonly shows BT or TT, but multibacillary disease can also present this way.

Borderline tuberculoid leprosy represents the peak of acute nerve damage (Fig. 4.22). The extent of pre-existing cellular infiltration makes the nerves extremely susceptible to damage from even minor degrees of acute inflammation during phases of reaction, which characterize all forms of borderline disease (instability peak). Fewer nerves are affected than in BB but the potential for rapid and permanent damage is much greater.

Untreated borderline tuberculoid leprosy can continue for many years. Bouts of reaction accelerate nerve damage and multiple deformities follow as a result of anaesthesia, muscle paralysis and

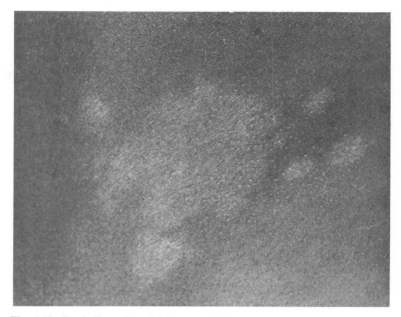

Fig. 4.19 Borderline tuberculoid leprosy (BT). This group of macules was the only cutaneous sign of leprosy but the right ulnar and great auricular nerves were also enlarged. Note the hypopigmentation, the rough surface and the marginal definition, but in places the edge is less distinct and there are satellite lesions which suggests that the patient's immune response is not quite containing the infection (BI 1+).

contracture. Many cases finally heal — 'the burnt out case'. Others downgrade with successive reactions and the disease becomes increasingly lepromatous, so that the complications of bacillary invasion are added to those of the already destroyed nerves.

Borderline lepromatous leprosy (BL)

Features here are a mixture of those attributable to bacillary invasion and those of the unstable centre of the spectrum.

Skin lesions resemble those of lepromatous leprosy, but on detailed examination a number of differences are found. The lesions are not distributed absolutely symmetrically on the body. Areas of apparently normal skin are found between the lesions. The lesions may differ from each other in size and shape. Papules and nodules may stand out clearly from the skin, rather than merging imperceptibly into an infiltrated background (Fig. 4.23, 4.24). Larger lesions, either macules or plaques

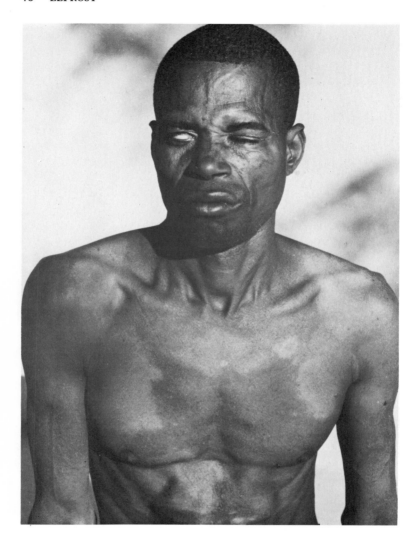

Fig. 4.20 Borderline tuberculoid leprosy (BT). This is the typical appearance of one form of BT leprosy (sometimes called low resistant tuberculoid) in which there are numerous widespread macules. Some macules are large enough to cover a whole limb, others are small and seem to coalesce. The macules are hypaesthetic, dry and hypopigmented. They do not develop into plaques. Despite the quiet appearance of the skin lesions, nerve damage is always extensive and type 1 reactions causing severe acute neuritis are common. AFB are scanty (BI 1–2). This patient has an early facial nerve lesion. He is trying to close his eyes and cannot approximate the right lids; lagophthalmos. There is seldom much weakness of the lower half of the face, in contrast with Bell's palsy and upper motor neurone lesions.

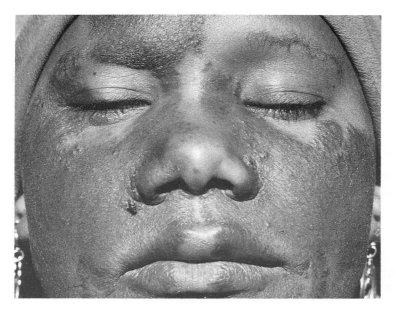

Fig. 4.21 Borderline tuberculoid leprosy. On paler skins, lesions are often red or copper coloured. This one is well-defined, irregular, pebbly and dry. In this case the colour has been enhanced by clofazimine which is preferentially taken up by the lesion in the skin.

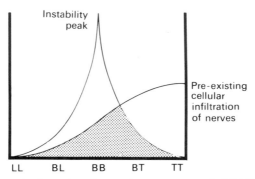

Fig. 4.22 The peak of severity of nerve damage, composed of liability to type 1 reactions in already infiltrated nerves in BT and BB leprosy. In this diagram the instability peak is exaggerated since it is instability which predisposes to reactions.

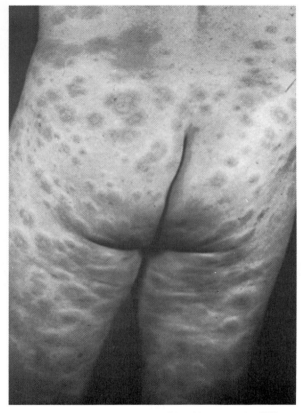

Fig. 4.23 Borderline lepromatous leprosy (BL). Numerous bacilliferous nodules and plaques are almost symmetrical bilaterally. A colour photograph would show the erythema in this pale skin. The spreading edges of many of the lesions suggest that the disease is downgrading.

in an asymmetrical distribution, or lesions with punched out centres, may suggest that the disease began much nearer the tuberculoid pole and then downgraded (Figs. 4.25, 4.26). Eyebrows are not completely lost.

Bacillary invasion of the nose and larynx are not as severe as in LL, and keratitis, lepromata of the eye, testicular atrophy and gynaecomastia do not usually develop unless the disease downgrades.

Anaesthesia will resemble that found in LL, but may lack complete symmetry; large peripheral nerves become thickened earlier than in LL with corresponding anaesthesia and paresis which, too, may not be

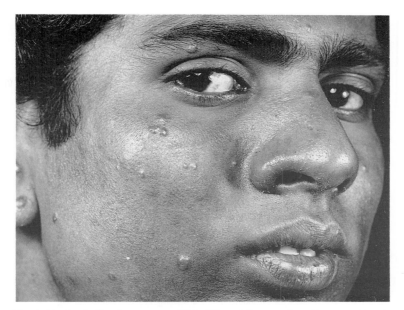

Fig. 4.24 Borderline lepromatous (BL). BL nodules are often discrete and well-defined, although the intervening skin is also heavily infected. Compare these circumscribed dome-shaped papules with the pointed papules and pustules of erythema nodosum leprosum in Figure 8.5.

symmetrical. Nerves are, however, unlikely to be damaged as quickly as in BB and BT leprosy.

BL leprosy represents the peak of rapid downhill progress, compounded of instability and bacillary multiplication (Fig. 4.27). The patient's disease is on the 'wrong' side of the instability peak and all too often downgrades towards LL with its attendant complications. Even so, clinical signs characteristic of the earlier borderline phase can probably be made out. Recognition of these signs is important, as they indicate that the patient has the potential to some cellular immunity, and type 1 reaction, the prognosis on treatment is better than in cases of LL that never exhibit borderline characteristics. In South-east Asia about 80% of lepromatous patients have some evidence of old borderline disease. The proportion is even higher in Africa.

Downgrading may be accompanied by inflammation of all the lesions, in which case the patient may be greatly distressed although nerve damage is not so serious as in patients with BT leprosy.

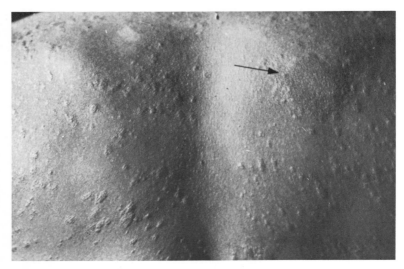

Fig. 4.25 Downgrading: BT–BL. A longstanding lesion of BT leprosy was present over the right scapula for nearly a year. The edges then became swollen and increased in extent although the central area of healing remained flat: this is a typical appearance of BB lesion (arrowed). At the same time innumerable small papules and nodules appeared all over the body, but especially the face and trunk. They are shiny, erythematous, of varying definition and tend to spare the midline of the back. Bacterial index in these lesions was 5+. In this case a mild type 1 reaction accompanied downgrading and most of the peripheral nerves were tender on palpation.

Extension of disease

Leprosy can get worse in two ways:

1. The disease spreads, but does not alter its clinical characteristics or its position on the spectrum. This is invariable and continual with untreated LL and can occur for varying times at other points on the spectrum.

2. A diminution in cell mediated immunity shifts the patient's position on the spectrum towards the lepromatous pole (downgrading), with corresponding changes in the characteristics of the disease. This happens in borderline disease. Downgrading may at first cause a reduction in features of disease activity, such as swelling and pain, and the patient's condition may deteriorate a long way before it is noticed.

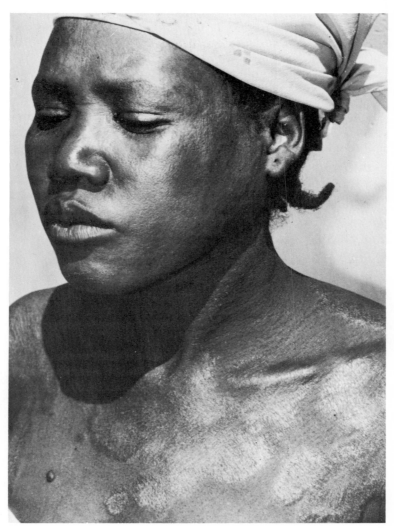

Fig. 4.26 Downgrading BT–BL. This patient was being treated in a leprosy clinic for typical BT lesions, which may be seen on her trunk. Because of type 1 reactions, which are evidenced by the raised edge and scaly surface of the lesions, her dapsone was reduced to an inadequate dose. She then developed iritis due to type 2 reactions, and close examination showed the diffuse infiltration of the face and loss of eyebrows characteristic of lepromatous disease.

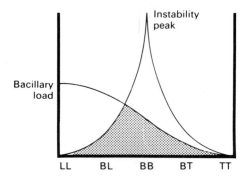

Fig. 4.27 The peak of rapid downhill progress, composed of liability to rapid downgrading and bacillary multiplication.

PROGNOSIS

The prognosis of untreated leprosy depends mainly on the patient's position on the spectrum (Fig. 4.28). At the lepromatous pole the patient gets steadily worse. The causes of death have already been listed (see p. 38). At the tuberculoid pole recovery is the rule, but anaesthesia and paralysis from individual nerve destruction may occur. Borderline disease (BL, BB, BT) will behave ultimately in one or other of these two

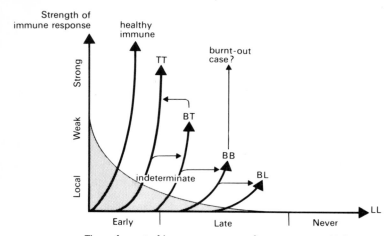

Fig. 4.28 Hypothetical scheme suggesting how the type of clinical disease may be affected by the time of onset of the immune response and by its strength. The hatched area represents subclinical disease (after Godal, 1972).

ways, but whichever way it goes, extensive deformity from multiple nerve damage will be likely.

Factors affecting prognosis

Treatment

Treatment improves the prognosis in two ways. First it stops bacillary multiplication, thus reducing the bacillary and antigenic load and preventing extension of disease. Secondly, in all patients other than those whose disease starts as pure LL it permits the re-emergence of, or an increase in, cellular immunity which shifts the patient's position towards the tuberculoid pole so that natural healing aids treatment and reduces the relapse rate. Without some degree of cellular immunity relapse will follow the cessation of treatment since it is impossible to kill the last single bacillus simply by treatment with the drugs available at present.

Race

Natural resistance varies. It appears to be greatest in the Negro, less in the Mongolian and least in the Caucasian. Indians, however, have a greater resistance than Anglo Indians, Burmese, Chinese and Europeans. The lower the resistance the greater the liability to develop lepromatous disease.

Age

Leprosy is usually an endemic disease. It is commonly acquired in childhood and self healing forms are usual. Of those who continue into adult life with leprosy there is therefore a greater proportion with poor resistance. The lepromatous rate is generally slightly higher in adults than in children, but the disease is not inherently worse in adults.

Sex

In most parts of the world, leprosy affects males more often than females, in the ratio of 2:1. But in some, especially African, countries the sex ratio is equal, or even reversed. Differences in sex ratio, which are more marked in adults than in children, may reflect exposure to infection rather than susceptibility to type of disease. Adult males, however, have a higher lepromatous rate than adult females and are liable to develop greater deformity.

Pregnancy

During pregnancy there are increasing levels of circulating corticosteroids, oestrogens and thyroid hormone and a non-specific depression of cellular immunity. In early pregnancy the normal T/B cell ratio is reversed (see Ch. 7). These changes are associated with reduced resistance to, especially, intracellular infections which may be reactivated. The changes are rapidly reversed in the puerperium, and resistance is regained. Pregnancy is liable to precipitate the appearance of leprosy for the first time, and of relapse. The disease may become worse as a result of downgrading, if not on treatment, or through the appearance of dapsone resistance, if on monotherapy (see Ch. 6). Type 2 reactions are common during the first trimester and during lactation, and type 1 reactions are common in the puerperium, associated with upgrading. These reactions may cause sudden nerve damage (see p. 118). Puberty, especially in girls, is associated with similar though less severe risks. Babies born to lepromatous mothers have low placental and birth weights, gain weight slowly after weaning, and are susceptible to marasmus and intercurrent infection.

Rate of progress of disease

The prognosis is worse in patients whose disease is rapidly progressive than in those whose disease has been relatively inactive for a long time.

Malnutrition and intercurrent infection

Although it is known that malnutrition in young children may lower resistance to several infections, no association has been shown between malnutrition and the incidence or type of leprosy. Leprosy patients may become malnourished and this could slow their recovery. Intercurrent infections, such as cellulitis, osteomyelitis and tuberculosis worsen the prognosis in several ways (see Ch. 9).

FURTHER READING

Barton R P E 1974 A clinical study of the nose in lepromatous leprosy. Leprosy Review 45: 135–144
Browne S G 1974 Self-healing leprosy: report on 2,749 patients. Leprosy Review 45: 104–111

Browne S G 1984 Leprosy. In: Acta Clinica Ciba-Geigy: S.A. Basle

Duncan M E 1985 Leprosy and procreation — a historical review of social and clinical aspects. Leprosy Review 56: 153–162

Godal T, Mykleslud B, Samuel D R, Myruang B 1971 Characterisation of immune defect in lepromatous leprosy. A specific lack of circulating *Mycobacterium leprae* — reactive lymphocytes. Clinical and Experimental Immunology 9: 821–831

Hansen G A, Looft C 1895 Leprosy: its clinical and pathological aspects. Transl. Walker N, Reprinted 1973 Wright, Bristol

Karat S, Karat A B A, Foster R 1968 Radiological changes in bones of the limbs in leprosy. Leprosy Review 39: 147–169

Liu Tze-Chun, Qui Ju-Shi 1984 Pathological findings on peripheral nerves, lymph nodes and visceral organs of leprosy. International Journal of Leprosy, 52: 377–383

Martin F I R, Maddocks I, Brown J B, Hudson B 1968 Leprous endocrinopathy. Lancet, 2: 1320–1321

Ortiz Y, Giner M 1978 Lucio leprosy (Diffuse lepromatous leprosy) II Recent advances: clinical and laboratory data. Dermatologia (Mexico City) 22: 141–163

Paterson D E, Job C K 1964 Bone changes and absorption in leprosy. In: Cochrane R G, Davey T F (eds) Leprosy in theory and practice. Wright, Bristol, pp 425–446

Pearson J M J, Ross W F 1975 Nerve involvement in leprosy. Pathology, differential diagnosis and principles of management. Leprosy Review 46: 199–212

Sabin T D, Ebner J D 1969 Pattern of sensory loss in lepromatous leprosy. International Journal of Leprosy 3: 239–248

Sehgal V N, Srivastrava G 1987 Indeterminate leprosy: a passing phase in the evolution of leprosy. Leprosy Review 58: 291–299

5. Diagnosis

The diagnosis of leprosy can usually be made by clinical examination supported by slit skin smears. Occasionally other investigations are necessary.

CARDINAL SIGNS OF LEPROSY

1. Anaesthesia. This may be of individual skin lesions or in the distribution of a large peripheral nerve, as in tuberculoid leprosy; or it may be over the areas of fine nerve involvement in lepromatous leprosy, beginning with the extensor surfaces of the forearms and legs, hands and feet.

2. Thickened nerves, at the sites of predilection (see p. 29).

3. Skin lesions. The essential characteristic of lesions of tuberculoid leprosy in a dark skin is hypopigmentation, whether they are macular or infiltrated. In a light skin the lesions are copper coloured or red. (Plates 1, 5)

4. Acid-fast bacilli in slit skin smears in lepromatous and borderline lesions.

At least two of the first three cardinal signs or the fourth should be present for the diagnosis of leprosy to be made.

HOW TO EXAMINE FOR LEPROSY

1. Take a history. This is often uninformative, but ask about numbness, the painfulness of recent burns or cuts, the evolution of skin lesions, difficulties in walking or grasping, eye trouble, family contact with leprosy, previous treatment with dapsone.

2. Strip the patient, naked if possible and stand him in a good, even, natural light. If in doubt try slanting sunlight; this helps demonstrate some lesions, but the intense shine from dark skins may make lesions difficult to see.

3. Look at the skin from afar and then closely for:

patches (macules or plaques), often hypopigmented. The vague early lesions of lepromatous leprosy are erythematous rather than hypopigmented.

nodules

infiltration

burns, scars, ulcers — especially of the hands and feet. Are they painful? Does the patient know how they happened?

4. Feel the nerves for enlargement and tenderness. Be gentle.

Ulnars. With the patient facing you, place your little fingers in the olecranon grooves and feel the nerve immediately above the groove with your other fingers. Feel for thickening, irregularity, hardness and tenderness and for difference between the two sides. Run your hands down the ulnar borders of the forearms and hands and feel for dryness of skin and wasting of hypothenar muscles.

Cutaneous branch of the radial. Roll it under your fingers as it crosses the lateral border of the radius just proximal to the wrist joint.

Median. Deeply, above or below the antecubital fossa, medial to the brachial artery, and deeply above and in front of the wrist between the tendons of palmaris and flexor carpi radialis.

Radial. Roll it in its groove on the humerus posterior to the deltoid insertion.

Lateral popliteal. With the patient facing you place your thumb on the upper border of the patella and with your fingers around the knee, feel the nerve in the popliteal fossa just medial to the biceps femoris tendon. The medial popliteal nerve may also be palpable here. Follow the course of the lateral popliteal nerve and roll it as it passes round the neck of the fibula.

Posterior tibial. This lies beside and deep to the posterior tibial artery as it passes posteriorly and inferiorly to the medial malleolus.

Anterior tibial. This emerges from under the flexor retinaculum lateral to the tendon of extensor hallucis longus and to the dorsalis pedis artery.

Great auricular nerve. Turn the head to one side, thus stretching the nerve across the sternomastoid. This nerve is often visible or palpable in a thin person.

Supraorbital. Run your index fingers across the forehead from the midline laterally. An enlarged nerve is palpable as it runs up out of the orbit.

Cutaneous nerves in relation to patches. The enlarged nerve may be proximal to the patch or deep to it, but rarely distal to it.

5. Test for anaesthesia. Using a wisp of cotton wool, touch normal skin to determine the level of normal sensitivity. Touch a spot once only. Do not stroke. Compare sensation in normal skin to that in a patch. Cotton wool may be too delicate for thickened skin on palms and soles, in which case use a leaf or piece of paper or a pencil point. Ask the patient to touch the place you touch, accurately, with the tip of a finger. When he can do this ask him to shut his eyes and continue. Inability to identify the point stimulated accurately is called misreference. It is the earliest sign of hypaesthesia. The normal range of accuracy is from 2 cm on the face to 7 cm on the back and buttocks. Test:

in relation to patches. Lesions of tuberculoid leprosy on the face may not always be hypaesthetic.

in relation to enlarged nerves and to the fifth cranial nerve, including the cornea.

over the extensor surfaces of the hands, forearms, feet, legs and buttocks.

over the rest of the body.

Test also for loss of sensation to pain (pin prick) and temperature (test tubes containing hot and cold water).

On the soles of the feet and palms of the hands test for light pressure, which is the protective sensation (ball-point pen or pencil).

6. *Look for complications*, lepromatous invasion of the eye, nose, larynx and testes.

reaction: tender nerves, erythema nodosum leprosum, irid-ocyclitis, orchitis, dactylitis, tenosynovitis.

sensory nerve damage: burns, cuts, ulcers, scars, loss of digits.

motor nerve damage: weakness, loss of muscle bulk and tone, paralysis, contractures (see p. 134 for signs of individual nerve lesions).

autonomic nerve damage: impaired sweating, decreased hair growth, peripheral cyanosis, poor capillary return.

7. *Complete a general clinical examination.*

8. *Acid-fast bacilli.* Make, stain and examine slit skin smears (see laboratory diagnosis below).

9. *Take a skin biopsy* if the diagnosis is still in doubt.

10. *Decide:*

a. Does the patient have leprosy?

b. If so, where does his disease lie on the spectrum?

c. What is the state of activity?

d. Is the patient having a reaction (see Ch. 8)?

e. Should more sophisticated, quantitative tests of nerve function be performed (see p. 136)?

f. What treatment should be given and for what:

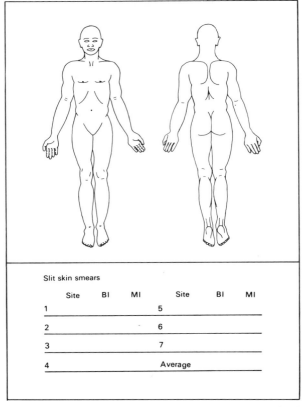

Fig. 5.1 On this chart are recorded the sites of skin lesions and of enlarged nerves, the pattern of anaesthesia and the results of slit skin smears.

specific anti-leprosy, anti-inflammatory, for complications of leprosy, or general for malnutrition or intercurrent illness?

g. What are the social implications of these decisions?

Clinical observations may conveniently be summarized on a body diagram (Fig. 5.1) and on a disability record (Fig. 5.2).

LABORATORY DIAGNOSIS

Slit skin smears

Smears are made from suspect lesions as well as from sites commonly affected in lepromatous leprosy, usually the earlobes, forehead, chin,

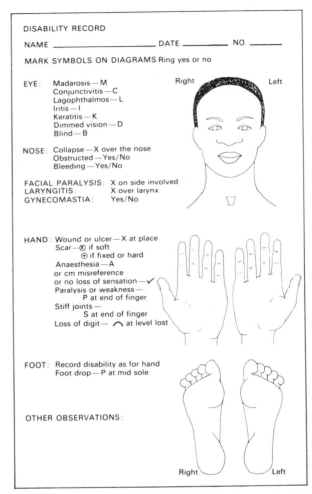

Fig. 5.2 Disability record. Careful completion of this chart at the initial examination ensures that the patient's disabilities are recorded, and treatment of them is not overlooked. At intervals during treatment a new chart is made out to help assess progress.

extensor surfaces of forearms, dorsal surface of fingers, buttocks and trunk.

The skin is cleaned with alcohol or ether. In light of the possibility of the patient being HIV positive, WHO recommends that gloves should be worn while taking smears. A fold of skin is picked up between finger and thumb and is squeezed tightly to prevent blood

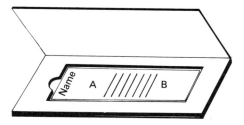

Fig. 5.3 Slide mailing tray prepared for making slit skin smears. A white card fixed in the bottom of the tray has lines marked on it. The slide is laid on the card and a smear is made over each of the lines. In reading heavily infected smears the objective needs to travel only from A to B.

flow. A small incision is made into the dermis with a small sharp sterile★ scalpel blade (preferably a Bard-Parker number 15). The blade is then turned through 90 degrees and used to scrape the cut surface of the tissue. The juice so obtained is smeared onto a slide and allowed to dry.

A bloody smear is valueless. Six to eight smears may be placed transversely on the same slide.

Standardization of slides is obtained by using a slide postal tray to hold the slide while smearing (Fig. 5.3). On the bottom of the tray is a white card on which six to eight parallel lines are marked and each site is smeared along a line in a set order. This aids in rapidity of examination as one movement of the stage across all the smears is often adequate to complete the bacillary index and morphological index.

A nasal smear is made from any site of infiltration in the nasal cavity. With the aid of a speculum and a good light the nose is carefully examined and the lesion scraped with a flattened probe or fine spatula.

In place of the standard nasal smear, a 'nose blow' smear examination is worthwhile. Nasal discharge or mucus is obtained by having the patient blow his nose in a piece of polyethylene plastic and immediately smearing the mucus, bloodstained if possible, on a separate slide. This is helpful not so much as a diagnostic procedure but, by estimating the morphological index, as a means of determining if the person is infectious.

★ A fresh disposable blade is preferred for each patient. Reused blades may transmit hepatitis B, HIV and other infections unless properly sterilized. The World Health Organization recommends sterilization of cleaned blades by autoclaving, boiling for 10 minutes, or disinfection for 20 minutes in 70% ethanol, formalin, or 1% chlorine-sodium hypochlorite.

The slide is flamed to fix the smear as soon as it is dry and stained by *Ziehl-Neelsen's method*. Leprosy bacilli are not quite as acid-fast as tubercle bacilli. A suitable modification of the method which avoids the necessity of heating the slide is:

1. Cover the slide with freshly filtered cold strong carbol-fuchsin/ Tween 80 and leave for 10 minutes.
2. Flood off the stain with water.
3. Cover the slide with acid-alcohol/methylene blue and leave for 3 minutes.
4. Wash well under the tap and blot dry.

Reagents are prepared as follows:

Strong carbol-fuchsin/Tween 80. 3.5 g basic fuchsin is dissolved in 12.5 g pure phenol with gentle heating. Cool and add 25 ml 95% alcohol or spirit. Make up to 300 ml with distilled water and add 30 drops Tween 80 *or* Teepol — other detergents might do equally well — and stir without frothing.

Acid-alcohol/methylene blue. 1 ml of concentrated hydrochloric acid is added to 100 ml 70% alcohol or spirit. Dissolve in this 0.6 g methylene blue.

The more usual carbol-fuchsin stain does not contain a detergent. Penetration of stain into the bacilli is assisted by heating the carbol-fuchsin covered slide to 60°C (until it steams, but without boiling) for 5 minutes before washing, decolourizing and counter-staining. This method may be more reliable when dealing with smears of low bacterial index. It also tends to produce a higher morphological index.

After staining, slides are examined using a 100× oil immersion lens. Bacilli are seen as red rods against a blue background. The presence of bacilli confirms the diagnosis of leprosy. The density of bacilli is recorded as the *Bacterial Index:*

6+ many clumps or over 1000 bacilli in an average field
5+ 100 to 1000 bacilli in an average field
4+ 10 to 100 bacilli in an average field
3+ 1 to 10 bacilli in an average field
2+ 1 to 10 bacilli in 10 fields
1+ 1 to 10 bacilli in 100 fields.

In advanced lepromatous leprosy the Bacterial Index is 5+ or 6+, and begins to fall after about one year of treatment. In untreated patients earlobes often yield the greatest number of bacilli. In treated patients the dorsal surfaces of the fingers are often the last site to become negative. The index decreases across the spectrum to 0 to 2+ in BT leprosy (Fig. 4.9). Slit skin smears are negative in TT leprosy. Slit skin smears can only detect bacilli present at a concentration greater than 10^4 per g of skin, and so cannot be used as a test of cure.

As important is the *morphological index*, which is the percentage of solid staining bacilli. Bacilli that stain irregularly or are beaded or fragmented are dead (see p. 192). The morphological index is a useful index of progress under treatment and changes more rapidly than the bacillary index. In lepromatous leprosy it falls from its starting point of about 5–20% to zero after five to six months uninterrupted treatment with dapsone, or after about five weeks with rifampicin. A morphological index that rises after having fallen indicates either that the patient has not taken or absorbed his drugs or that the bacilli have become resistant to them.

Histology

Skin biopsy is indicated if the diagnosis is in doubt, as it may be in indeterminate leprosy. Biopsy of a cutaneous nerve twig may confirm the diagnosis of neural leprosy in the absence of skin lesions. Skin biopsy is necessary for the accurate classification of leprosy and may be of use in distinguishing between downgrading and reversal in type 1 reactions (see p. 120) and between relapse and reaction after termination of treatment in borderline leprosy (see p. 88).

Biopsy material is best fixed in FMA fixative (40% formaldehyde 10 ml, mercuric chloride 2 g, glacial acetic acid 3 ml, water to 100 ml) for two hours and then transferred to 70% alcohol. Alternatively 10% formol saline buffered to pH 7.0 can be used. Fixed tissue may be mailed to a histopathology laboratory. Sections are usually stained with haematoxylin and eosin for histology, and by the Fite-Faraco method for bacilli.

Serodiagnosis

Specific serological tests for leprosy (see p. 107) now make it possible to identify:

1. People that have been infected with *M. leprae*. Most of these will not develop clinical disease.

2. People with early, subclinical, lepromatous leprosy, who have high titres of antibody to phenolic glycolipid I and arabino-mannan, and in whose serum and urine antigens of *M. leprae* may be detected.

These tests are proving useful in epidemiological studies and may find a place in control schemes, but have not yet been applied to clinical and differential diagnosis of leprosy.

SKIN TESTS

Lepromin test

(See p. 113 for definition and performance.)
This is *not* a diagnostic test for leprosy: many people who have never been exposed to infection with *M. leprae* (for example in England) have positive Mitsuda reactions. The test is positive in cases of TT and BT leprosy and so may be of some help in classification; it is negative in LL, BL and, usually, BB leprosy (Fig. 7.4). A positive test in a case of suspected indeterminate leprosy excludes the diagnosis of leprosy or indicates that the disease has become tuberculoid leprosy. It may be of use in assessing the direction of immunological shift in borderline leprosy.

Histamine test

The wheal and flare response to histamine is the end product of a local reflex which depends upon the integrity of sympathetic nerve fibres. If a hypopigmented patch is due to leprosy the response of the skin to histamine will be delayed, diminished or absent.

A drop of 0.001% histamine acid phosphate is placed on the suspect lesion and another drop is placed on normal skin. The skin is pricked with a needle through each drop and the timing, intensity and extent of the flare which appears during the next ten minutes is recorded. In dark skins this test may be difficult to read.

Pilocarpine test

Sweating is dependent upon the integrity of parasympathetic nerve fibres. If a hypopigmented patch is due to leprosy the response of the sweat glands to a cholinergic drug will be diminished.

Inject 0.1 ml of 0.06% pilocarpine intradermally into the patch and into a normal control site. The sweat response is assessed visually, or more accurately by the conversion from white to blue of quinizarin powder which is retained on the test areas by strips of transparent adhesive tape. If quinizarin is not available the test area can be painted with tincture of iodine and allowed to dry before injecting pilocarpine and then dusted with starch powder; sweating turns the powder blue. The histamine and pilocarpine tests are seldom needed.

A simpler and more practical test is to exercise the patient in the sun and see if the patch sweats or not.

DIFFERENTIAL DIAGNOSIS

The diagnosis of leprosy should be made positively. The diagnosis should not be made by exclusion or by therapeutic trial. If the diagnosis is in doubt the lesion is either too early (indeterminate leprosy) or it is not leprosy. Strictly, therefore, confusion should arise only over macular lesions, but leprosy in all its stages can mimic a great variety of other conditions, of which the commoner ones should be known.

Local artefacts

In order to avoid making stupid mistakes the doctor should be familiar with local practices which may increase the difficulty in diagnosing leprosy.

Local attitudes. Do social circumstances lead people to hide leprosy, so that cases tend to come late? Do people bring any minor skin lesion to the attention of the doctor in the hope of getting dapsone for its antimalarial effect?

Normal range of skin colour. What is the range of skin colour and texture? Is it too dark for erythema ever to be visible? Many Africans have a distinct line of demarcation between pale ventral skin and dark dorsal skin along the upper arms and occasionally thighs. This could be mistaken for the edge of a large macule. Babies in harsh climates commonly have mottled cheeks.

Local occupations. Digging, hoeing, pounding and grinding each produce characteristic patterns of callus on the hands. These should not be mistaken for scarring of an anaesthetic hand. In Iran young girls who knot carpets at home have a characteristic deformity: the third finger of the right hand and to a lesser extent the fourth finger of the left hand are deformed as a result of forcible passage through the strong tight warp threads. This is not the result of an ulnar nerve lesion.

Local medical practices. What are they with regard to leprosy? In parts of Africa early leprosy lesions are cauterized with a hot iron. In parts of South-east Asia they are burnt with a paste made of lime, charcoal and alcohol. Each method produces a characteristic scar which can be recognized. A distinct patch of hypopigmentation around the scar, indicating spread since treatment, is almost diagnostic of leprosy. Cautery can never cure leprosy as the bacillus is already in the nerves.

Local cosmetic practices. Some animistic peoples deform their children in a variety of ways so that the spirits shall not be jealous of their beauty. Eyebrow plucking, amputation of the terminal phalanx of the little finger and filing of upper central incisor teeth, which may later fall out, are examples which could in isolation, be mistakenly considered signs of leprosy. Tattoos occasionally come to be surrounded by a halo of hypopigmentation, or even by a defined plaque with a tuberculoid histology. Tattooing has also been known to transmit leprosy (see p. 206). Fine multiple tribal scarifications can at first glance resemble lepromatous macules, and small dense keloids lepromatous nodules.

Common local skin diseases: dyspigmentation or keratitis in onchocerciasis, palmar hyperkeratosis from yaws producing contracture, or ringworm. Remember that hypaesthesia can accompany any hyperkeratotic lesion and that hypaesthesia of facial patches in leprosy is much less marked than on the trunk.

Two or more diseases often occur together. Patients with tinea versicolor, onchocerciasis (Fig. 5.4) or cutaneous leishmaniasis may get leprosy and the lesions in the skin may at first sight be confusing. Occasionally leprosy may co-exist with a rare skin disease.

Macular lesions

Babies commonly have blotchy cheeks, especially if they are exposed to sun and wind. Some blotches may be nutritional in origin, and other signs of protein and vitamin malnutrition should be sought. Some may be fungal.

Birthmarks are usually, but not always present from birth. Some may fade slowly over the years, but characteristically they do not alter their appearance, while untreated leprosy alters continuously. Birthmarks often have irregular, sometimes bizarre shapes and may show a variety of degrees of hypopigmentation in the same lesion. The edge is usually distinct, but the texture and character of the skin is otherwise normal.

Vitiligo. Complete loss of pigment is never due to leprosy. Vitiligo is characterized by depigmented macules of any size or shape, in any distribution; its cause is unknown. Complete loss of pigment may also follow lesions of endemic syphilis, yaws, onchocerciasis, burns or contact with certain chemicals.

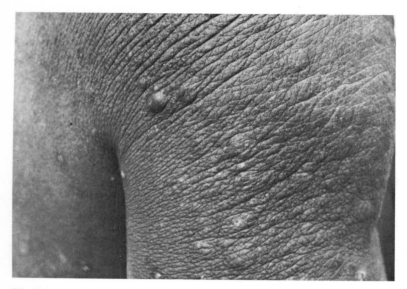

Fig. 5.4 Onchocerciasis. Chronic onchocerciasis produces either atrophy of the skin, in which case the skin hangs down in folds especially over the lower back and groins, or hypertrophy and nodulation of the skin as shown here. The distribution over the thighs, buttocks and shoulders and the absence of AFB distinguish the condition from lepromatous infiltration.

Fungal infections commonly mimic leprosy. The commonest is *Tinea versicolor* (tinea flava, tinea furfura, pityriasis versicolor) (Fig. 5.5). The lesions are usually small, smaller than lepromatous macules and numerous. They may be slightly hypopigmented, hyper-pigmented or erythematous and are covered in white floury scales. Individual lesions are discrete with clear edges, but often they fuse to cover large areas of skin. They are most commonly found on the upper part of the trunk and around the neck, and spread down the midline of the chest and back, the so-called necklace.

Seborrhoeic dermatitis also has a powdery surface in it milder forms. It usually starts on the scalp (dandruff), and spreads around the hairline, behind the ears and thence onto the trunk. Isolated lesions on the cheek might arouse a suspicion of leprosy, but careful inspection of the eyebrows and hairline is likely to reveal the typical changes. Pityriasis alba is characterized by round or oval, scaly, hypopigmented macules on the face and trunk of children, especially in Africa, and may simulate leprosy. The lesions resolve spontaneously in a few months. (Fig. 5.6).

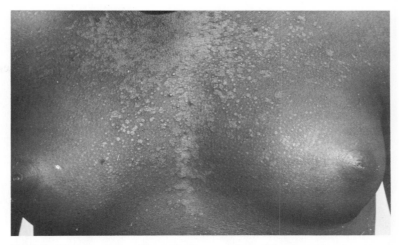

Fig. 5.5   Tinea versicolor. The white floury surface of these macules almost makes the lesions look like plaques. The small discrete macules are typical but they often coalesce and appear to flow down the back or chest, as in this picture, like a necklace. They are usually confined to the trunk, are not anaesthetic and do not contain AFB. Scrapings soaked in 10% potassium hydroxide show hyphae and spores.

Resolving inflammatory lesions of whatever cause (especially fungal infections, eczema, impetigo and pityriasis alba) are often surrounded by vague hypopigmented halos. A careful history may elicit their origin.

Plaques and rings

The commonest mimics of plaque-like lesions in leprosy are also diseases in whose pathogenesis cellular immunity or hypersensitivity are important and largely determine the clinical picture.

Ringworm. This fungal infection is often, but not always, in an area of skin which is warm and moist and often spared in leprosy. The raised edge is often inflamed and may contain vesicles or crusts which are never present in leprosy. Ringworm usually itches. Microscopic examinations of skin scrapings soaked in 10% potassium hydroxide to dissolve keratin should reveal characteristic hyphae. Treatment with topical fungicidal ointments will rapidly clear up most lesions.

Granuloma multiforme (Fig. 5.7). This is a disease of tropical Africa. It mainly affects adults who develop circinate lesions of varying size, often resembling tuberculoid leprosy. Most lesions have

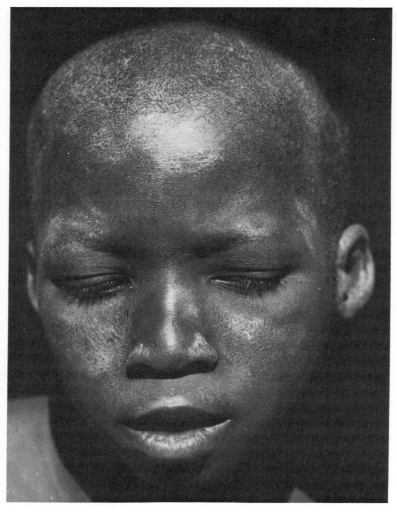

Fig. 5.6 Seborrhoeic dermatitis. This is the typical picture: a child with dry, scaly, hypopigmented macules affecting the cheeks, alae nasae, eyebrows, hairline and scalp. Similar lesions were present behind his ears and on his chest and upper arms. The clinical distinction from indeterminate leprosy may be difficult when there is only one such lesion, on the cheek or trunk.

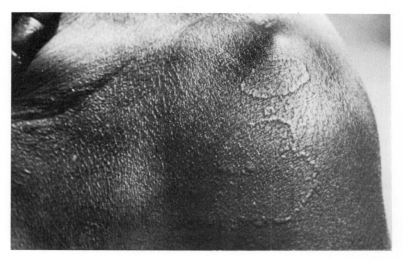

Fig. 5.7 Granuloma multiforme. The lesions are of normal pigmentation, have normal sweating and hair growth and are not anaesthetic. Differentiation from TT leprosy may be difficult (see Fig. 4.3), but histological examination shows that nerves are spared.

a fine infiltrated border, but without much hypopigmentation. Plaques are sometimes seen. They are distributed mainly over the upper part of the body, on face, trunk and arms. The lesions show no impairment of sensation or sweating. The lesions may remain static, change slowly or heal spontaneously. The aetiology is unknown.

Sarcoidosis. Skin lesions of sarcoidosis may be impossible to distinguish on sight from those of tuberculoid leprosy, but the lesions are not anaesthetic. There may be signs of systemic disease, or erythema nodosum. The Kveim test is positive.

Cutaneous tuberculosis (lupus vulgaris). Commonest on the face and assuming a great variety of clinical forms, this disease can usually be distinguished from tuberculoid leprosy by the greater extent of tissue destruction and the presence of scars in which can be seen small red or orange nodules. The lesions tend to heal at one edge and spread from another, rather than heal centrally as in leprosy.

Lupus erythematosus. Early lesions across the nose and cheeks may be raised, resembling a tuberculoid plaque, before atrophy and scarring begin; but unlike leprosy, there is follicular plugging.

In all these conditions the peripheral nerves are normal. Histology may be uninformative for, except in the case of lupus erythematosus, it will reveal a tuberculoid granuloma. The presence of normal nerve fibres within the granuloma would exclude the diagnosis of leprosy.

Other common dermatoses. *Lichen simplex* presents with plaques on the back of the neck and extensor surfaces of the arms and legs. The lesions itch and become thickened as a result of scratching. *Psoriasis* is rare in Africans, but common in Caucasians. It presents its typical appearance of pink plaques or circinate lesions covered with white scales which may be scratched away to reveal small bleeding papillae. *Lichen planus* presents in several ways: the commonest is of multiple small plaques, whose flat tops are covered with fine creases. Large grey nodules or hyperpigmented macules are other presentations. In these conditions the peripheral nerves are spared, and histological examination is helpful.

Nodules

Cutaneous leishmaniasis (Fig. 5.8). In the Savanna belt of Africa south of the Sahara, in North Africa and Ethiopia, in India and the Middle East, and in South and Central America cutaneous leishmaniasis is common. Depending upon the local epidemiological situation lesions may be either single or multiple. They are commonly on the face or arms. The lesion presents as a nodule which, after some months, ulcerates and heals (oriental sore). It may resemble tuberculoid leprosy if central healing is accompanied by slow peripheral extension (lupoid or recidivans leishmaniasis), or lepromatous leprosy if lesions fail to heal and new nodules appear, especially on the face where the distribution is like that of leprosy. This last condition (diffuse cutaneous leishmaniasis), which is seen in Ethiopia and South America, represents a failure of cellular immunity, and is therefore analogous with lepromatous leprosy. Slit skin smears do not contain acid-fast bacilli, but do contain amastigotes of *Leishmania*, which can be demonstrated by Leishman's stain. In some countries where kala azar occurs, notably India and Kenya, similar cutaneous lesions are sometimes seen after treatment (post kala azar dermal leishmaniasis).

Others. Nodules on the face, which might at first sight be confused with those of leprosy, are sometimes seen with neurofibromatosis, molluscum contagiosum, blastomycosis and histoplasmosis. Kaposi's sarcoma commonly arises in hands and feet (Fig. 5.9). The nodules are often deeply situated and bleed easily if injured. Their distribution and the absence of acid-fast bacilli exclude the diagnosis of leprosy.

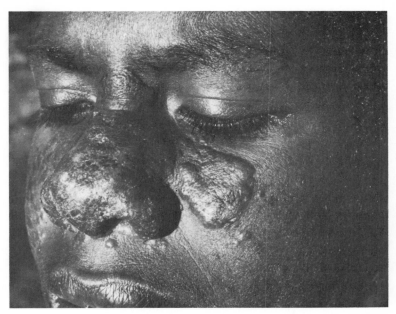

Fig. 5.8 Cutaneous leishmaniasis. This is an early case of diffuse cutaneous
leishmaniasis in an Ethiopian. The disease has spread locally from the primary
lesion on the bridge of the nose. The lesion is a plaque with distinct edges and
some satellite lesions. It might be mistaken for tuberculoid leprosy, but the
friable surface, which indicates a partial immune response, and predilection for
the mucocutaneous border of the nose are characteristic of leishmaniasis. Slit skin
smears stained with Leishman's stain revealed *Leishmania*. No nerves were enlarged.

Nerve lesions

Thickened nerves. For practical purposes, leprosy may be
considered as the only cause of thickened nerves in countries where it
is endemic. Other causes of thickened nerves are extremely rare, and
include:

1. Peroneal muscular atrophy (Charcot-Marie-Tooth disease) of
which the most common form is peripheral neuropathy inherited as an
autosomal dominant. Distal weakness and wasting dominate the
picture, tendon reflexes are lost and pes cavus is common. Nerve
biopsy is characteristic.

2. Dejerine-Sottas disease is a slowly progressive mixed peripheral
neuropathy, inherited as an autosomal recessive, starting in childhood.

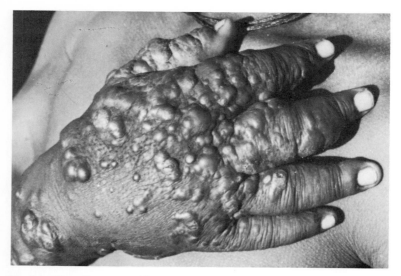

Fig. 5.9 Kaposi's tumour. The gross nodular swelling was confined to one hand and forearm. The tumour in this case arises deep in the tissues causing swelling of the whole hand. The rest of the body was normal. Profuse bleeding on slit skin smearing and the absence of AFB exclude leprosy. Histology is diagnostic.

The protein content of cerebrospinal fluid is raised. Nerve biopsy is characteristic.

3. Refsum's disease is similar to Dejerine-Sottas disease, but is commonly associated with other physical abnormalities and an accumulation of phytanic acid in the blood and tissues.

4. Nerves may be thickened in amyloidosis.

Anaesthesia may follow nerve damage due to trauma, local nerve compression or other causes of peripheral neuritis, in which case paraesthesiae or pain are usually also present. The peripheral neuritis which is associated with cassava eating in West Africa is often accompanied by signs of ataxia and optic atrophy. Syringomyelia is characterized by symmetrical anaesthesia to pain and temperature, but not to touch (dissociated anaesthesia). There are often lower motor neuron signs in the arms and upper motor neuron signs in the legs. Nerves are not enlarged.

Contractures. Dupuytren's contracture affects initially the fourth finger, congenital flexion deformity the fifth finger only, tertiary yaws the third, fourth and fifth fingers. These patterns and the absence of corresponding sensory loss exclude an ulnar or median nerve lesion.

Plantar ulcers may develop in any sensory neuropathy. They are particularly common in diabetes and in the dominantly inherited sensory neuropathy, whose onset is usually in the second or third decade. Nerves are not enlarged in either disease. Fissures of the feet are common in dry climates, and are normally painful; in wet climates they may be due to late yaws.

Eye lesions

Entropion and trichiasis are more commonly caused by trachoma than by leprosy.

Iridocyclitis and its complications have many causes. In endemic areas, leprosy and onchocerciasis are the commonest.

If in doubt, wait and observe. Do not treat for leprosy unless the diagnosis is established. Nothing is harder to cure than leprophobia. A mistaken diagnosis may cause severe social complications.

FURTHER READING

Aguado Sanchez C, Malik A, Tongue C, Lambert P H, Engers H D 1986 Simplification and standardization of serodiagnostic tests for leprosy based on phenolic glycolipid-I antigen. Leprosy Review 57 (suppl. 2): 83–93

Browne S G 1983 The diagnosis and management of early leprosy. The Leprosy Mission, London

Clarke G H V 1969 Skin diseases in the African. H K Lewis, London

Guinto R S, Abalos R M, Cellona R V, Fajardo T J 1983 An atlas of leprosy. Sasakawa Memorial Health Foundation, Tokyo

Jacyk W K 1983 Leprosy in Africans. German Leprosy Relief Association, Würzburg

Jones R L, Ponnighaus J M 1982 The transport of histological specimens by air mail. Leprosy Review 52: 67–68

Lechat M F, Misson C B, Walter J 1987 OMSLEP Recording and reporting system for leprosy patients. 3rd edition World Health Organization, Geneva

Leiker D L, McDougall A C 1983 Technical guide for smear examination for leprosy by direct microscopy. Leprosy Documentation Service (INFOLEP), Royal Tropical Institute, Amsterdam

Leiker D L, Nunzi E 1985 Leprosy in the light skin. Associazione Italiana "Amici di Raoul Follereau", Bologna

McLeod J G 1975 Peripheral neuropathy. Medicine, 2nd Series: 2197–2207

Ridley M J, Ridley D S 1971 Stain techniques and the morphology of *Mycobacterium leprae*. Leprosy Review 42: 88–95

Ridley D S 1977 Skin biopsy in leprosy. Documenta Geigy, Basel

WHO Guidelines for skin smears 1987. International Journal of Leprosy 55: 421–422

6. Treatment

Leprosy and its complications produce a wide range of disorders, and their management involves different disciplines of medicine, ranging from psychotherapy to reconstructive surgery. This chapter is concerned only with medical treatment of the uncomplicated infection. Management of complications is dealt with under Management of Reactions (Ch. 9), Physical Rehabilitation (Ch. 12), Social, Psychological and Vocational Rehabilitation (Ch. 13) and The Eye (Ch. 11). Until 1941 there was no really effective antileprotic, although Hydnocarpus oil, which had been used in India and China for centuries, was of some value.

Now several good drugs are available. The minimum inhibitory concentration that is required, and the plasma level that is achieved are known for most of them, and the rates at which they kill bacilli have been determined. Some properties of the most commonly used drugs are listed in Table 6.1. If these drugs are used correctly, and at an early stage of the disease, the prognosis is excellent. Since the recognition of drug resistance, and the development of the mouse footpad technique with which to study it (see p. 192), much theory and dogma have been published about the approach to leprosy treatment and control. However, the principles for the combined use of drugs have become clear and multidrug therapy (MDT) is now widely practised in the field. The results of on-going trials and of individual experience may yet be expected to modify the way these drugs are used.

DRUGS AVAILABLE

Sulphones

Sulphones were first used in treating leprosy in 1941, and they still remain the most useful drugs. Diaminodiphenyl sulphone (dapsone, DDS) was first synthesized in Germany in 1908, and was found to be

Table 6.1 Characteristics of drugs available for the chemotherapy of leprosy. (From WHO Study Group 1982)

Drug	Minimal inhibitory concentration (MIC) (μg/ml)	Dosage (mg)[d]	Ratio of peak serum concentration to MIC[a]	Number of days during which peak serum concentration exceeds MIC[b]	Bactericidal activity	Estimated cost ($/year)
Dapsone	0.003	100	500	4–12	low	0.60
Rifampicin	0.3	600	30	1	high	9.00 (1×mo)
Clofazimine[c]	?	50	?	?	low	13.50
Ethionamide	0.5	375	60	1	intermediate	60.00
Prothionamide	0.3	375	40	1	intermediate	60.00

a. Ratio of peak serum concentration in man, after a single dose, to MIC determined in the mouse.
b. Serum concentration in man after a single dose.
c. Because of uneven tissue distribution, estimate of the MIC is impossible.
d. Dosage in a $\geq$50 kg adult.

successful in controlling bacterial infections in experimental animals, but it proved to be too toxic in equivalent doses in man. In the late 1930s a substituted derivative of dapsone, glucosulfone sodium (promine) was found to have antituberculous activity in guinea pigs. For this reason, in 1941, Guy Faget tried it on patients with leprosy at Carville in Louisiana by daily intravenous injection and it was effective. Later Robert G. Cochrane used dapsone in oily suspension intramuscularly as a depot with success. In 1947 John Lowe in Nigeria tried the parent compound orally, but in much smaller doses, and found it was possible to avoid the extreme toxicity which had accompanied its early use.

Dapsone has proved to be cheap, safe and effective and eminently suitable for outpatient care, but since 1965 two major problems have emerged: dapsone resistance and microbial persistence.

Pharmacology

Dapsone is bacteristatic but its exact mode of action is not known. It is a competitive inhibitor of para-aminobenzoic acid and interferes with folate metabolism, but the unique sensitivity of *M. leprae* to dapsone suggests that some other mechanism may also be involved.

The minimal inhibitory concentration of dapsone in mice infected with *M. leprae* is 0.003 μg per ml. Dapsone is excreted exponentially and its half life in man is about 24 hours, with a range of 13–40 hours in different individuals. A single dose of 100 mg in man gives a blood level of about 1.5 μg per ml, which is weakly bactericidal and which falls to the minimal inhibitory concentration in 4–12 days. Very small doses of dapsone (1–10 mg per day) give bacteristatic blood levels above the minimal inhibitory concentration but encourage the emergence of resistant strains and should not be used.

The morphological index of bacilli from smears of patients with lepromatous leprosy treated with dapsone falls to zero in five to eight months.

Administration and dosage

Dapsone is commonly made up in 100 mg tablets. In some countries other sizes are available. Dapsone should be given as a single daily oral dose of 50 mg or 100 mg for an adult and 2 mg/kg body weight/day for a child. If the patient's reliability is in doubt dapsone can be given by intramuscular injection of 600 mg weekly. Dapsone should normally be given with one or more other antileprosy drugs (see p. 86).

The repository compound, acedapsone (4,4 diacetyl-diaminodiphenyl sulphone, DADDS) releases dapsone, or its monoacetylated derivative very slowly, and an injection of 225 mg given every 75 days produces a satisfactory initial response and has been tried in large scale programmes (see, p. 224). Its routine use is not recommended because plasma levels are much lower (0.02– 0.1 μg per ml) than with standard oral dapsone, and could encourage the emergence of resistant strains of *M. leprae*.

Side effects

These are rare when dapsone is used in the currently recommended daily doses. They can be considered as:

1. Dose dependent

Acute psychosis, which is rare.

Anaemia. Mild haemolysis is common but severe anaemia is rare and usually occurs in association with intercurrent infection and glucose 6-phosphate dehydrogenase deficiency. If severe anaemia develops another drug should be used instead of dapsone.

Hypoalbuminaemia and neuropathy leading to muscular weakness have been reported in patients taking very large doses of dapsone for other skin diseases.

2. Idiosyncratic

Allergic rashes including exfoliative dermatitis which can be fatal. The onset is usually one to two months after starting treatment and may be accompanied by fever and jaundice.

Fixed drug eruption, often appearing as hyperpigmented or black macules.

Agranulocytosis has been reported as a result of taking 25 mg daily for malarial prophylaxis but this was in addition to other drugs.

3. Due to death of bacilli and liberation of bacillary antigens

Any effective antileprotic drug can trigger off a reaction (see p. 115) and dapsone does this most frequently as it is used most frequently. Some patients therefore, particularly borderline patients in the early stages of treatment and lepromatous patients after some months or years, appear to become intolerant of dapsone.

In the past, treatment of patients was often begun at a low dose for fear of precipitating reactions. Now, it has been shown clearly that the severity and incidence of type 2 reactions in lepromatous leprosy are not affected by the dosage of dapsone.

Resistance

In the past 25 years dapsone resistance has become an increasing problem around the world. Most resistance has been secondary, appearing in multibacillary patients after 10–20 years of treatment with dapsone alone. The delay in the appearance of resistance from 1945 to 1965 may have been due to the weakly bactericidal levels produced by conventional dosage of dapsone. Primary resistance began to appear in the late 1970s and is rarer. It is due to infection with dapsone resistant *M. leprae* and may present in patients with any type of leprosy. The degree of resistance may be low, intermediate or high, as measured by the dietary dose of dapsone needed to inhibit replication in the mouse footpad (see p. 192).

Prevalence rates of secondary dapsone resistance in multibacillary patients treated for over 5 years vary widely, but are approaching 100% in Ethiopia, Shanghai and parts of India. Most of this resistance is of high degree. The incidence of secondary resistance ranges from 0.1% in Malaysia to 3% in Ethiopia and Mali. Primary dapsone resistance is usually low or intermediate and prevalence rates range from 3% of new patients in the Philippines to over 50% in China, Ethiopia, and Nepal. Most patients would be expected to respond clinically to dapsone given in full dosage. Rates of high degree resistance are under one-tenth these figures. This means that dapsone is still a useful drug in MDT regimen.

Secondary dapsone resistance may be suspected when a patient with LL or BL leprosy, who has been on dapsone monotherapy for many years, develops new active lesions. In the skin, the lesions may have characteristics different from those of the original infection. They may present as isolated firm nodules (histoid leprosy), which resolve poorly with the new drug, or they may arise de novo as large succulent nodules on a restricted area of skin such as one arm, or the back. Occasionally they are more widely dispersed over the body. The face usually continues to have the wrinkled appearance of inactive disease, and smears from it and from the ears have low bacterial and morphological indices while the new lesions have indices of 5+ to 6+ and 50% respectively. Bacilli in these new lesions are often uniform in appearance. Resistance may also be suspected if a long treated patient with quiescent disease unexpectedly develops a type 2 reaction.

Resistance may be confirmed clinically or experimentally. The patient is given regular and supervised dapsone in full dosage for six months. If, at the end of this time, the morphological index has not fallen near to zero, resistance is confirmed. Where laboratory facilities exist, bacilli should be tested for dapsone sensitivity into the mouse footpad (see p. 195).

Persistence

Separate from the problem of resistance is the observation that viable *M. leprae*, fully sensitive to dapsone, can be isolated from nerves, smooth muscle and striated muscle in approximately 50% of lepromatous (BL, LL) patients who have taken dapsone un-interruptedly for óver 10 years, and who show no signs of active disease. These bacilli are capable of multiplying once treatment is stopped and causing a clinical relapse. It is postulated that persisters are dormant bacilli and thus escape the action of drugs. Unfortunately no drug or combination of drugs has yet been found that will eliminate persisters.

Rifampicin

Rifampicin (Rifadin) is the most effective anti-leprosy drug and brings down the morphological index in lepromatous leprosy to zero in about five weeks. It is given orally in a dose of 600 mg once daily, or 450 mg for patients weighing under 35 kg. Although bacteria are rapidly killed, the rate of fall of the bacterial index, the speed of the clinical improvement and the incidence of type 2 reactions in lepromatous patients are the same as with dapsone. Rifampicin has two drawbacks. It is very expensive, and it may produce toxic syndromes. Its toxicity depends both on the dosage (renal failure and hepatitis being more frequent with large doses) and on the interval between doses (fever, haemolytic anaemia and thrombocytopenia being more frequent when the drug is given at weekly intervals). No toxic effects have been reported with monthly administration.

It has been shown that daily administration of 600 mg of rifampicin is no more effective than monthly administration of 600 mg on each of two consecutive days. Because of its expense and the risk of toxicity, treatment with rifampicin should be fully supervised.

Rifampicin has not proved to be a quick cure for leprosy. Persisters can still be found in preferred sites in lepromatous patients who have been treated with rifampicin daily for 5 years. But it does render lepromatous patients non-infectious within 2 days, and is the mainstay of MDT regimens (see p. 86). Rifampicin resistance is so far rare, but the drug should never be prescribed on its own. It is not recommended in the first trimester of pregnancy.

Aminoglycoside antibiotics

Streptomycin is bacteristatic against *M. leprae*. In the past it was found to be effective against lepromatous ulceration of the face and nasal septum, but it has now given way to rifampicin. It is a useful second line drug, given in an adult dosage of 1 g daily, or 20 mg/kg body weight for a child, by intramuscular injection. Used on its own, resistance develops rapidly. In mice streptomycin has an additive or synergic effect when given with rifampicin.

Kanamycin is effective against *M. leprae* in mice, but has not yet been used in man.

Clofazimine

This substituted iminophenazine dye (Lamprene-Ciba Geigy; B-663) is unique in leprosy, as it has an action equal to that of dapsone and also an anti-inflammatory effect which is of value in reactional states. Clofazimine is a red crystalline substance which is suspended in an oil/wax base and marketed in gelatin capsules of 50 and 100 mg. The drug is best absorbed after food and is distributed unevenly in tissues, high concentrations being reached in intestinal mucosa, lymph nodes and fatty tissue. The serum half life is about 10 days but the tissue half life may be as long as 70 days. A steady state is reached after about six weeks. Because of the uneven distribution, its MIC cannot be calculated. Resistance to clofazimine is very rare: the drug has been used on its own for many years to treat dapsone resistant patients. Its precise mode of action is not known, but it probably interferes with mycobacterial DNA.

The adult dose for the treatment of leprosy infection (as opposed to reaction) is 50 mg daily or 100 mg thrice weekly, and for children 1 mg/kg/day. In control schemes, monthly doses may also be given (see p. 87). In this dosage clofazimine reduces the frequently of type 1 and type 2 reactions by almost 30%. When given to treat reactions, a higher dose is given (see p. 130).

The drawbacks of clofazimine are its cost, the development of skin pigmentation and abdominal symptoms. The skin first becomes red, then brown and eventually blue-black. This pigmentation varies with the initial skin colour, and leprosy lesions pigment more deeply than normal skin. The conjunctivae become red, and the urine, sputum and sweat pink. Fat is dyed orange, and viscera brick red. The lighter the initial skin colour, the more objectionable is the pigmentation. However, even Caucasians, if they have suffered prolonged reactional states, find the colour preferable to the misery. For darker skinned persons the pigmentation is acceptable. Itching, dryness and cracking of the skin occur frequently but are not problems. Crystals of clofazimine are deposited in the small bowel mucosa and mesenteric lymph nodes. Nausea and diarrhoea can often be controlled by giving the capsules with food. High doses of clofazimine can cause severe abdominal pain. Persisting viable bacilli have been found in lepromatous patients treated for 6 years with clofazimine.

Clofazimine is recommended as part of the regimen for the treatment of multibacillary leprosy. It may be used to treat dapsone resistant leprosy. It is also of value in patients who are to undergo surgery (see p. 176), or have reactions involving the eye.

Ethionamide and prothionamide

Ethionamide and prothionamide are virtually interchangeable (see Table 5.1), and show cross-resistance to each other. These two thioamides are effective bactericides in the recommended dose of 5–10 mg/kg/day. Experimental studies in mice suggest that the bactericidal activity of these drugs is compromised if not given daily. They are more expensive and more toxic than dapsone. There is a significant threat of hepatotoxicity, so determination of serum transaminase should be made prior to and every 2 to 4 weeks during therapy. At the dose of 10 mg/kg/day the degree of toxicity is quite unacceptable. At the lower rate of 5 mg/kg/day this is reduced to 10–20%. Even so, a proportion of patients become jaundiced, especially in China and other parts of Asia. Hepatotoxicity seems to be more of a problem when the drug is administered with rifampicin. Due to their toxicity the thioamides drugs are the least desirable of the choices of bactericidal drugs for oral use.

Thiourea compounds

Thiacetazone

Thiacetazone (thiosemicarbazone, p-acetaminobenzaldehyde) is the only one still available. It is cheap and may be useful as a second line drug. It is given orally in a dose of 150 mg daily. Leprosy bacilli develop resistance to it rapidly and are then cross-resistant to ethionamide.

TREATMENT REGIMENS — MULTIDRUG THERAPY (MDT)

In 1982, following the deliberations of a study group, the World Health Organization drew up specific recommendations for treating leprosy with more than one drug.

Rationale and principles of MDT

Experience in the treatment of tuberculosis had shown that the problem of drug resistance could be overcome by using a combination of at least two effective drugs. Both drugs kill or prevent the multiplication of sensitive organisms, and each drug prevents the growth of organisms resistant to the other. In a population of $M. leprae$, one organism in 10^6 will show low degree resistance to dapsone, one in 10^{10} high degree resistance to dapsone and one in 10^7 resistance to rifampicin. Low dose or irregular treatment and monotherapy encourages the growth of these mutants.

Patients with paucibacillary leprosy harbour less than 10^6 viable $M. leprae$ and have good cell mediated immune responses; the use of two drugs should be adequate to prevent the emergence of resistance. Patients with multibacillary leprosy harbour 10^{9-10} viable $M. leprae$, out of a total 10^{11} organisms, and have no cell mediated immune response. Mutants resistant to two drugs will be present; so three drugs may be needed to prevent the emergence of resistance (Fig. 6.1).

One or two doses of rifampicin kills 5 log organisms, reducing the load of live $M. leprae$ to 10^4 in multibacillary disease, and eliminating most or all mutants resistant to dapsone and clofazimine. This leaves 10^4 rifampicin sensitive organisms, which is too few to give rise to further resistant mutants, and 10^2 rifampicin resistant organisms, which should be killed by six months treatment with dapsone and clofazimine. Some organisms will survive as persisters, in theory for up to 7 years. Two years treatment should produce relapse rates under 1%, and with drug sensitive organisms.

Rifampicin, being bactericidal, may be given monthly, which is once every two divisions of $M. leprae$. Dapsone, being bacteristatic and with a short half life, must be given daily. Clofazimine has a depot effect, but monthly dosage is not adequate; however, a monthly supplement to daily or alternate day dosage will ensure adequate levels if compliance is poor.

The regimen recommended for MDT is a compromise between theoretical ideals and goals achievable under field conditions in poor countries.

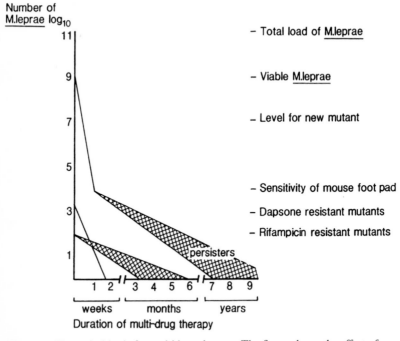

Fig. 6.1 Theoretical basis for multidrug therapy. The figure shows the effect of treatment on the bacterial load of a patient with advanced lepromatous leprosy who may be expected to harbour 10^{11} organisms, of which 10^9 are viable. One or two doses of rifampicin kills 5 $\log_{10}$ organisms, including all dapsone resistant mutants, within a few days. Dapsone, or clofazimine, kills all rifampicin resistant mutants in a few months. Persisters remain viable for many years, but should be fully sensitive to all three drugs in the event of relapse.

MDT regimens:

Paucibacillary leprosy. For the purposes of MDT, this includes patients with indeterminate, TT and BT leprosy, with some exceptions that are treated as multibacillary patients. Adult patients should receive:

> rifampicin 600 mg once monthly, supervised and
> dapsone 100 mg once daily, unsupervised

Treatment is given for six months.

Multibacillary leprosy. For the purposes of MDT, this includes:

> 1. Patients with BB, BL and LL leprosy.

2. Patients with more than 15 skin lesions or widespread nerve involvement regardless of classification: these patients may exhibit episodes of bacillaemia.

3. If histology is not available, patients whose slit skin smears show *any* acid-fast bacilli (it is easy to misclassify borderline patients on the results of slit skin smears).

4. Relapsed multibacillary patients regardless of any change in classification.

Adult patients should receive:

> rifampicin 600 mg once monthly, supervised and
> dapsone 100 mg daily unsupervised and
> clofazimine 50 mg daily supervised and
> clofazimine 300 mg monthly, supervised.

Treatment is given for two years, or 24 months in a 36 months period, or until smear negative, but never for less than 24 months. The thioamides are used if drug intolerance develops or if clofazimine is refused on cosmetic grounds.

These regimens are now widely accepted, although local variations may be found, for example some prefer to give rifampicin on the first two days of each month. Some ignore 'until smear negative' and treat every patient with multibacillary disease for 24 months, regardless. Some treat paucibacillary disease for 12 months.

Surveillance after treatment

When chemotherapy has been completed, patients with paucibacillary disease are seen every six months for two years and with multibacillary disease for at least five years. Patients are questioned and examined for evidence of activity or reactivity, and slit skin smears are carried out on multibacillary patients.

Benefits of MDT

If properly implemented, MDT

1. Prevents drug resistance.
2. Treats pre-existing dapsone resistant infection.
3. Eliminates the need to determine the sensitivity of *M. leprae* before starting treatment.
4. Shifts the concept of treatment from prolonged treatment that merely arrests the disease, to a short course of treatment that cures the disease. By boosting morale this

5. Increases compliance — in some schemes from 50% to 95%.
6. Prevents deformity more efficiently.
7. Halves the case load each year.
8. Renders patients non-infectious more quickly.
9. Reduces the long-term costs of control programmes.

Problems with MDT

1. Case definition. Clinical assessment and slit skin smears will misclassify a proportion of multibacillary cases as paucibacillary and result in undertreatment and inadequate follow-up, especially in patients with widespread BT leprosy in whom biopsies may show many more acid-fast bacilli in nerves than in skin. The technique of slit skin smears is not uniformly practiced or interpreted. This makes it difficult to compare the results of trials from different places.

2. Disease activity. At the end of six months treatment the clinical signs in many patients with paucibacillary leprosy will not have resolved, although the bacilli are dead. Doctors as well as patients may be unhappy to stop chemotherapy. This is a serious problem in India, where up to 30% of paucibacillary patients remain clinically active. Treatment may be continued for a further six months, although the benefit of this has not been proven; 80% clinical cure rates at the end of treatment in paucibacillary leprosy converts to over 95% in 3–4 years.

3. Reaction or relapse? Reactions accompanying reversal may occur up to three years after starting treatment in paucibacillary patients, and many years later in BL or subpolar lepromatous patients. New nerve lesions may appear, and in BL patients who upgrade new skin lesions are common. The distinction between relapse and reaction may be difficult, even with the aid of histology. If chemotherapy has only recently been completed, treatment for the reaction alone is given. If the reaction does not settle quickly or if treatment has been stopped over a year ago, or slit skin smears show solid bacilli, chemotherapy is also resumed.

4. Relapse. About 2–3% paucibacillary patients may be expected to relapse after 6 months MDT. In one study in India 12 months treatment with rifampicin and dapsone reduced the relapse rate to zero. Relapse occurs within the first two years after stopping treatment, and is commonest in lepromin negative patients (who may have been misclassified), in patients with numerous lesions, and in young women. The relapse rate in multibacillary disease after MDT does not seem to be any higher, which is encouraging as half the relapses may be expected in the first three years after stopping treatment. Experience with dapsone monotherapy showed a cumulative relapse rate of 9% over 20 years, so the true relapse rate with MDT is not yet known. Wherever possible, drug sensitivity of relapse organisms should be determined in the mouse footpad.

5. Persisters. MDT does not eliminate persisters. After two years their number has been calculated at about 10^4 in a lepromatous patient. Relapses due to multiplication of persisters should be drug sensitive.

6. Operational aspects of MDT are considered in Chapter 16.

IMMUNOTHERAPY

Attempts to reverse the immune defect of lepromatous leprosy are still in the experimental stage. Local injection of heat-killed *M. leprae* with BCG may bring about a local cell mediated reaction that clears bacilli from that site. Repeated injections, which may cause painful ulcers, may induce a more general reversal and trigger reactions. Similar results have been claimed for other myobacteria, used similarly. At the moment these methods have no place in treatment. Some experimental workers have claimed to reverse the immune defect in vitro, by the addition of interleukin 2, or other mediators, (p. 103) to lymphocyte cultures, but there is no general agreement on these results and they are not applicable to patients.

MANAGEMENT OF PATIENTS

Outpatient programme

Most patients with leprosy are managed in outpatient clinics. Where skilled staff are scarce and supervision poor the standard of care may be far from ideal, but outpatient clinics alone can reduce the incidence of deformity greatly and this must be one of the aims. One of the factors limiting the efficacy of outpatient clinics on their own is that treatment may precipitate a reaction and so cause anaesthesia and paralysis.

If pain or tenderness develops in a nerve the leprosy attendant should refer the patient to hospital at once, or if that is not possible, should splint or rest the affected limb and treat with such antiinflammatory drugs as may be available, including steroids. Chemotherapy is continued.

It should be stressed to all paramedical workers, and to those supervising outpatient programmes, that anaesthesia, paralysis and other disabilities resulting from acute neuritis are not inevitable consequences of leprosy, and referral to a leprosy hospital is urgent whenever they threaten. Patients should be examined regularly for evidence of progressive nerve dysfunction or tenderness.

An essential part of any leprosy programme is the education of patients as to the doses of drugs and the duration of treatment, the safe-keeping of their tablets, the recognition of reaction and the prevention of injuries and disability. This is an additional effort for staff but is an investment that will reap untold benefits if carried out with enthusiasm and with an approach acceptable to the patients.

In hospital

Many patients will benefit from a short stay in hospital at the start of their treatment. There are several reasons for this:

1. The patient can be properly examined by the doctor, who may not have time to visit outpatient clinics often enough.
2. The most suitable type of treatment can be started.
3. The routine of regular treatment is established.
4. Reactional states can be diagnosed and controlled.
5. Early disability can be detected and treated.
6. Intercurrent illness can be treated.
7. The patient is taught to protect an anaesthetic hand or foot.
8. The patient can learn from those who have already benefited by education and acknowledge their anaesthesia.
9. The patient has an opportunity to become acquainted with the hospital in case future care is required.

Every effort should be made to help the patient who has social, psychological or occupational problems. The patient is taught that with regular attendance and care he need not become disabled or deformed.

FURTHER READING

Almeida J G et al 1983 The significance of dapsone (DDS) resistant *M. leprae* in untreated patients. International Journal of Leprosy 51: 374–377
Baohong J I 1985 Drug resistance in leprosy — a review. Leprosy Review 56: 265–278
Baohong J I et al 1984 Hepatotoxicity of combined therapy with rifampicin and daily prothionamide for leprosy. Leprosy Review 55: 282–289
Cartel J L et al 1985 Hepatotoxicity of the daily combination of 5 mg/kg prothionamide and 10 mg/kg rifampicin. International Journal of Leprosy 53: 15–18

Ellard G A 1984 Rationale of the multidrug regimens recommended by a W.H.O. Study Group on chemotherapy of leprosy for control programmes. International Journal of Leprosy 52: 394–401

Huikeshoven H 1983 Compliance and compliance testing. Health Cooperation Papers 1: 83,63–68. Organizzazione per la Cooperazione Sanitaria Int., Bologna

Jesudasan K, Christian M 1985 Risk of paucibacillary leprosy patients released from control relapsing with multibacillary leprosy. International Journal of Leprosy 52: 19–21.

Jesudasan K, Christian M, Bradley D 1984 Relapse rates among non-lepromatous patients released from control. International Journal of Leprosy 52: 304–310

Jopling W H 1983 Side effects of antileprosy drugs in common use. Leprosy Review 54: 261–270; also 1985 56: 71–73

Jopling W H et al 1984 A follow-up investigation of the Malta-project. Leprosy Review 55: 247–253

Kaur S, Sharma V K, Kumar B 1984 Treatment of leprosy — newer concepts. Indian Journal of Leprosy 56: 307–312

Kumar A 1984 Treatment compliance by leprosy out-patients and its monitoring under field conditions. Indian Journal of Leprosy 56: 313–318

Leiker D L, Nunzi E 1984 Leprosy in the light skin. Organizzazione per la Cooperazione Sanitaria Int., Bologna

McDougall A C 1988 Implementing multidrug therapy for leprosy. Oxfam Practical Guide No. 3. Oxford, England

Nunzi E (ed) 1983 Management of leprosy in countries with developed health services. Health Cooperation Papers, Organizzazione per la Cooperazione Sanitaria Int., Bologna, Italy

Pattyn S R 1984 Incubation time of relapses after treatment of paucibacillary leprosy. Leprosy Review 55: 115–123

Pattyn S R et al 1984 Hepatotoxicity of the combination of rifampicin — ethionamide in the treatment of multibacillary leprosy. International Journal of Leprosy 52: 1–6

Pearson J M H 1983 Dapsone resistant leprosy. Leprosy Review — Special Issue: 85S–89S

Rees R J W 1982 An appraisal of medical research in the treatment and control of leprosy. Leprosy in India 54: 783–800

Schaad-Lanyi Z, Dieterle W, Dubois J-R, Theobold W, Vischer W 1987 Pharmacokinetics of clofazimine in healthy volunteers. International Journal of leprosy 55: 9–15

Touw-Langendikj E M J, Naafs B 1979 Relapses in leprosy after release from control. Leprosy Review 50: 123–127

Warndorff van Diepen T, Aredath S P, Mengistu G 1984 Dapsone-resistant leprosy in Addis Ababa: A progress report. Leprosy Review 55: 149–157

WHO Expert Committee on Leprosy 1988 Sixth Report. Technical Report Series 768. World Health Organisation, Geneva

WHO Study Group 1982 Chemotherapy of leprosy for control programmes. Technical Report Series 675. World Health Organization, Geneva

Yawalkar S J, Vischer W A eds 1984 Lamprene (clofazimine) in leprosy: basic information. Ciba-Geigy Ltd., Basle

7. Immunology

The response of the body to invading microorganisms involves both specific and non-specific mechanisms of defence. Non-specific mechanisms include the barriers of skin and mucosae, antisepsis of sebum and mucosal secretions, acidity of gastric juice, production of acute phase proteins, activation of the alternative pathway of complement, natural antibodies, fever, and simple phagocytosis and digestion by polymorphonuclear leucocytes and macrophages. Specific mechanisms are those elaborated by the immune response. They contribute to healing and immunity, hypersensitivity and pathology. Successful parasites, such as *M. leprae*, have developed ways to avoid or subvert these mechanisms.

BASIC IMMUNOLOGY RELEVANT TO LEPROSY

A microorganism consists of and produces many different chemical substances which are antigenic. These antigens reach the lymphoid organs (lymph node or spleen) where each is potentially capable of inducing an immune response. The type of response induced is determined by the nature of the antigen, the way in which it is presented to lymphocytes, and the cellular events that follow.

Immune response

The immune response to most organisms has two components, cellular and humoral. Cell mediated immunity is mediated by lymphocytes that are processed in fetal life by the *thymus*, and are referred to as T-lymphocytes or T-cells. Humoral immunity is mediated by By-lymphocytes or B-cells and their progeny, plasma cells, which secrete antibodies. In birds B-lymphocytes are processed in the *bursa* of Fabricius, an organ associated with the hind gut and having no anatomical equivalent in mammals. In man B-lymphocytes are processed by the bone marrow.

93

The response is regulated by a complex set of humoral and cellular 'feedback' mechanisms that ensure its orderly build-up, progression and decline when no longer needed. Thus there are many stages at which the immune response may be suppressed or deviated.

Immune tolerance is the most extreme form of suppression, and may occur by one of several mechanisms. There may be a genetically inherited non-responsiveness to a particular antigen, or an acquired deletion or loss of function of T-lymphocytes specific for the antigen. By contrast there may be non-specific suppressions caused by suppressive factors released from cells or by selective removal of stimulatory factors. When the immune response is paralysed by an antigen specific mechanism, subsequent challenge with the same antigen fails to elicit any response. T-lymphocytes are required for both cell mediated and humoral immunity, so that suppression of T-lymphocytes may affect both arms of the immune response. In lepromatous leprosy, however, patients are able to produce antibodies but no cell mediated response to *M. leprae*.

Changes in lymphoid tissue

A schematic lymph note is shown in Fig. 7.1. During the course of an immune response certain changes take place in the lymph node which receives the antigen, or in the spleen in the case of circulating antigens. Antigen from an intradermal site is presented by macrophages which enter through the marginal sinus and pass between the germinal

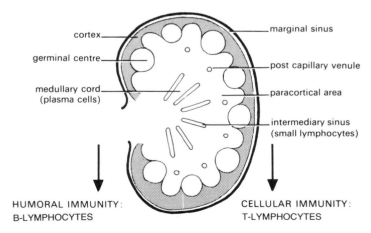

cortex

germinal centre

medullary cord
(plasma cells)

marginal sinus

post capillary venule

paracortical area

intermediary sinus
(small lymphocytes)

HUMORAL IMMUNITY:
B-LYMPHOCYTES

CELLULAR IMMUNITY:
T-LYMPHOCYTES

Fig. 7.1   Schematic lymph node.

centres into the paracortex. After this the parts of the node which develop depends upon whether humoral or cellular immunity is induced.

Humoral immunity. The cortex expands and germinal centres increase greatly in number and size, often bulging into and distorting the rest of the node. Plasma cells appear in the medullary cords which become thickened. In a pure antibody response the paracortex is thinned. Histological staining with pyronin, which stains ribonucleic acid red, shows the intense activity of germinal centres and medullary cords. These changes are seen in lepromatous leprosy.

Cellular immunity. The paracortical area of the node, whose development is dependent upon the integrity of the thymus in fetal life, expands. It becomes populated by small lymphocytes, which enter through the postcapillary venules, and start to divide. These large pale dividing cells are also pyroninophilic on staining. Small non-pyroninophilic lymphocytes are produced and leave the node through the intermediary sinuses, which become greatly distended. In a pure cell mediated response the cortex and medulla are thinned. These changes are seen in tuberculoid leprosy.

Most micro-organisms contain antigens which between them elicit both types of response.

Antigens

The antigens of *M. Leprae* are discussed in Chapter 2 (see p. 7 and Table 2.1). The following comments apply to properties of antigens in general.

Chemical nature. Some antigens, especially polysaccharides and simple chemicals (haptens) with a poor affinity to host proteins, are only weakly antigenic, especially with regard to cellular immunity. *M. leprae* is rich in polysaccharides, which may become split off their parent protein or lipid.

Molecular size. Substances, including some proteins, of low molecular weight (below about 10 kd) are often poorly antigenic, and are liable, under certain circumstances, to induce tolerance. Polymers of these substances and molecules of high molecular weight are more immunogenic. *M. leprae* has antigens around and below this size.

Concentration. A very high concentration of antigen may induce tolerance rather than immunity. In an already immunized host such a concentration may suppress the expression of cellular immunity (desensitization), producing a situation similar to immune deviation. This mechanism may underlie the process of downgrading in borderline leprosy. Patients with multibacillary disease have high concentrations of antigen, especially phenolic glycolipid in all infected tisues, and in plasma and urine. A very low concentration of antigen may also be tolerogenic.

Solubility. A highly soluble antigen is more likely to achieve a high circulating concentration and be less immunogenic than a poorly soluble antigen, or one that complexes with host proteins.

Route of presentation to lymphoid tissue. Antigens may reach the lymphoid tissue through the blood stream or along the lymphatics. They may be free or taken up by macrophages. Poorly soluble antigens, inoculated intradermally, phagocytosed by macrophages and taken by the lymphatics to the regional lymph node are highly immunogenic, especially with regard to cellular immunity. This is probably the case when *M. leprae* is inoculated through the skin. Antigens absorbed from the gut tend to induce immune suppression. Highly soluble antigens circulating free in the bloodstream are much less efficient in inducing immunity, especially cellular immunity, and may be liable to induce tolerance. *M. leprae* prefers to multiply in the Schwann cells of peripheral nerves. This is a privileged site because the organisms are intracellular and do not induce expression of class II molecules (see below), and because there are no lymphatic vessels in the perineurium. Antigens secreted by *M. leprae* probably pass directly into the venous blood, and reach the spleen where, if they are of suitable nature and concentration, they might suppress rather than induce cellular immunity.

Adjuvants. Certain substances, notably the cell wall lipids of *Mycobacteria*, have the property of augmenting both the humoral and cellular immune response to a wide range of antigens inoculated in emulsion with the adjuvant. Cell walls of *M. leprae* probably act as efficient adjuvants.

The HLA system and antigen presentation

The outcome of infection in man is, at least in part, under genetic control. Genes influence infection at two points. The first is immediately after infection when genes may determine whether the organism can multiply in man and so establish the disease, for example whether an essential substrate is available for a particular intracellular parasite. The second point is soon after the infection has been established and determines the host response to the infection, and thus influences the pattern and outcome of the disease. When a single gene is involved, the association with disease may be clear, as with ankylosing spondylitis and HLA-B27. But often many genes are involved, their inheritance is complex, and numerous other factors influence the outcome of infection. Then it is difficult to identify the genetic control. In leprosy one group of genes, situated in the HLA complex, has been associated with the outcome of infection with *M. leprae* (p. 211). But the HLA complex has a much more fundamental role in infection because it determines the manner in which antigen is presented to lymphocytes and thus controls the induction of the immune response, especially of cell mediated immunity. It also 'restricts' the interaction of lymphocytes to certain types of cell, which carry on their surface molecules, or 'gene products', produced on instruction by an HLA gene. The complex of genes, their products and their interaction with T-lymphocytes is known as the HLA-system. HLA (human leucocyte antigen) products are also the tissue transplantation antigens.

HLA genes are situated, like a string of beads, on the short arm of chromosome 6 (Fig. 7.2). They are divided into two classes. Class I contains (HLA-) A, B, and C genes. Class II contains three groups of genes (HLA-) DP, DQ, and DR. Each gene has many different possible variants or 'alleles', which gives the HLA system its enormous variability or polymorphism, and accounts for the wide range of human resistance and susceptibility to infection. (An allele is to a gene as a substitute is to a player in a particular position in a football team.) The genes control the production of certain glycoprotein molecules, which form part of the cell membrane and may be 'expressed' on the cell surface. Class I molecules are expressed by most nucleated cells and class II molecules by immunocompetent cells, i.e. B-cells, activated T-cells and antigen presenting cells (monocytes, macrophages dendritic cells and Langerhans cells). Schwann cells do not express class II molecules.

T-lymphocytes will only recognize antigen that is 'presented' in association with an HLA molecule on the surface of an antigen presenting cell. Cytotoxic T-lymphocytes (Tc cells, see p. 101) recognize class I molecules and so are able to act against a wide range of cells, such as tumour cells and virus infected cells. Regulatory T-lymphocytes (T-helper cells, TH), and possibly some T-suppressor cells, Ts) recognize class II molecules, so their interactions are restricted to immunocompetent cells. Some gene products, depending on the allele, promote efficient T-cell functions, others produce a poor T-cell response or no response and contribute to susceptibility to the organism. The terms immune response (Ir) and immune susceptibility (Is) are sometimes applied to these genes.

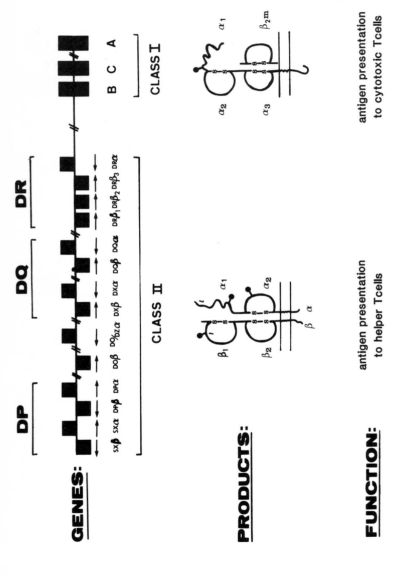

Fig. 7.2 Schematic representation of the HLA system (after Ottenhoff & de Vries, 1987)

In leprosy, HLA-DR molecules are needed to present *M. leprae* antigens to reactive T-lymphocytes. As a result TH cells proliferate: so HLA-DR is an Ir gene for *M. leprae*. However, Ts cells may also proliferate, presumably as part of the normal control system. DR3 is also associated with tuberculoid leprosy and lepromin positivity. One other HLA gene, DQwl, may by contrast be an Is gene for leprosy as it is associated with lepromatous leprosy and lepromin negativity.

Antigen presentation without HLA molecules

Figure 7.3 shows that free antigen is capable of stimulating B-cells and suppressor T-cells. It is possible that, in individuals who do not express HLA-DR efficiently, soluble antigens of *M. leprae* induce a form of immune suppression by stimulating T-suppressor cells and antibody production, which could permit the development of lepromatous leprosy.

Induction of the immune response

Antigen brought to lymphoid tissue, and correctly presented, sensitizes T- and B-lymphocytes of the appropriate clone that has the specific receptor site on their surface. This triggers a complicated cascade of cellular interactions which are mediated by soluble products (cytokines) of monocytes (monokines) and lymphocytes (lymphokines).

The study of these events, which are still imperfectly understood, has been made possible by the availability of monoclonal antibodies: antibodies produced from a single clone of B-lymphocytes that recognize only a single antigen or epitope. Many different monoclonal antibodies have been made use of, and the antigens they recognize on lymphocyte surfaces do not necessarily correlate with that cell's function (Table 7.1).

B-lymphocytes

Immunoglobulin D receptors on the surface react with free antigen and divide several times to produce plasma cells which secrete specific antibody, in one or more immunoglobulin class. Some antigens require help from TH cells to trigger B-lymphocytes. B-memory cells are also produced. In a primary immune response IgM antibodies are normally produced first, then IgG. IgM circulates as a pentamer, and is efficient at clearing the circulation by producing large complexes with antigens to

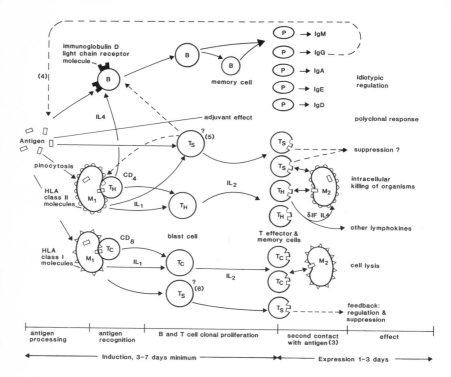

Fig. 7.3 Interaction of cells, lymphokines and antibodies in the induction, expression and regulation of the immune response.

1. Solid lines represent activation or progression, dotted lines suppression.

2. B = B-lymphocyte, P = plasma cell, Ig = immunoglobulin, M_1 = macrophage or other antigen presenting (e.g. dendritic) cell, M_2 = macrophage or other phagocytic cell capable of presenting antigen, T_H = T-helper cell, T_S = T-suppressor cell, T_c = cytotoxic cell.

3. Persistent contact with antigen (or repeated contact as in secondary immune response), causes (i) further interleukin 2-dependent proliferation of T_H lymphocytes; (ii) further proliferation of T_S cells; (iii) the production of more plasma cells. These stages are omitted here for clarity.

4. IgG antibody complexed with antigen regulates further antibody production. In addition anti-idiotype antibodies may suppress T_H cell function.

5,6 The existence of a CD4 suppressor cell and the suppressive role of CD8 cells are not proven.

organisms which are removed by phagocytosis. But it penetrates tissue poorly. IgG antibodies penetrate inflamed tissues well and opsonise or kill free organisms, but not intracellular organisms. IgA antibodies prevent organisms from adhering to mucosal surfaces. No protective role has yet been shown for antibodies in leprosy, though IgA and IgG antibodies *could* play a role in protection against reinfection.

Table 7.1 T-lymphocyte subsets relevant to leprosy: a simplified guide

Clusters of differentiation	Monoclonal antibodies	Functional characteristics
CD 1	OKT 6	Thymocyte and Langerhans cells
CD 2	Leu 4, OKT 11	Pan T-cell
CD 3	Leu 1, OKT 3	Pan T-cell
CD 4	Leu 3, OKT 4	T-helper
CD 8	Leu 2, OKT 8	T-suppressor
CD 8	Leu 2, OKT 8	T-cytotoxic

CD are clusters of cells differentiated by monoclonal antibodies, and do not necessarily distinguish function. Hence the uncertainty regarding the role e.g. of OKT 8 positive cells in the lesions of tuberculoid leprosy.

T-lymphocytes

T-helper cells (CD4, Table 7.1) react with antigen and Class II HLA molecules on an antigen presenting cell and become activated. This stage requires the monokine interleukin I which is secreted in response to phagocytosis or pinocytosis. The activated TH cell secretes the lymphokine interleukin 2. TH cells have receptors for interleukin 2, which in the presence of antigen will cause them to divide and so create a population of effector cells and memory cells. Memory cells persist to initiate secondary immune responses. TH cells cooperate with B-lymphocytes by producing the lymphokine interleukin 4 (B-cell growth factor).

Cytotoxic T-cells (CD8) react with antigen and Class I HLA molecules on an antigen presenting cell, are activated and undergo division in much the same way as TH cells. The activated Tc cell, sometimes known as a killer lymphocyte or Tk cell, kills certain tumour cell and virus infected cells in the presence of antibody.

Suppressor cells (Ts) suppress TH activity. In vitro CD8 cells have this property, and some workers suggest that CD4 cells contain a population of suppressor cells. Such cells might act by killing TH cells or by 'mopping up' available lymphokines needed for TH proliferation. In addition macrophages may suppress TH activity through the production of prostaglandin. The role of suppressor cells in regulating the responses in tuberculoid leprosy and suppressing responses in lepromatous leprosy, is hotly debated, but not settled.

Natural killer cells. These lymphocytes (NK cells), are not activated immunologically. They kill tumour cells and virus infected cells without antibody. No role for these cells has been postulated in leprosy.

Expression of immune response

Humoral immunity (antibody mediated)

There are several ways by which antibody can help the body to get rid of microorganisms. At the same time 'unwanted' responses to many of the antigens induce a state of hypersensitivity which contributes to the pathology of the disease.

The most important of these mechanisms are:

1. Antibody combines with and neutralizes toxins, as in diphtheria or typhoid, but probably not in leprosy.

2. Circulating antibody (opsonizing or complement fixing) reacts with antigen on the wall of the organism. In the first case rapid and efficient phagocytosis ensues. In the second complement is fixed and the organism is lysed. Neither of these mechanisms seems to be important in defence against leprosy.

3. Antibody passively coats host cells and is available to react with antigen. This antibody is of one of two kinds. It may be cytophilic for macrophages, in which case that cell is better enabled to take up microorganisms; this mechanism may be important in cell mediated immunity to certain facultative intracellular organisms, but it does not increase the digestive power of that macrophage, and may not be relevant in leprosy. Alternatively the antibody is reaginic of the class IgE and is fixed to mast cells. Circulating antigen reacts with the fixed antibody giving rise to the phenomena of local or systemic anaphylaxis. This does not seem to happen in leprosy.

4. Precipitating antibody combines with antigen, which is present in moderate excess, and forms complexes to which complement is fixed. This may take place either in the circulation or in the tissues. Complexes formed in the circulation are deposited, depending on their size, in the endothelial spaces of vessels, notably those in the glomerulus, the skin and synovial membranes. A depot of antigen, in the tissues, such as a lepromatous nodule, can be the origin of a gradient of antigen concentration. Antibody diffuses from the circulation and at the appropriate relative concentrations complexes are formed and deposited. Complement is fixed and the release of its activated third and other components attracts polymorphonuclear leucocytes which accumulate, phagocytose the complexes and release enzymes, of which the most potent are proteases which cause tissue damage. Activation of

vascular endothelium further encourages adhesion of leucocytes and platelets, thrombosis and haemorrhage. This process is important in the genesis of type 2 reactions in leprosy.

Cell mediated immunity (lymphocyte and macrophage mediated)

Antibodies do not normally penetrate host cells. Certain organisms have become adapted to intracellular life, and those which are adapted to intramacrophage life are especially well protected. These organisms include *Leishmania, M. leprae, M. tuberculosis*, certain fungi and, to a lesser extent, the more facultative intracellular organisms, *Salmonella* and *Brucella*. Cellular immunity is of especial importance in dealing with infections caused by these organisms. It is also of importance in some viral infections, in graft rejection and in tumour immunity.

There are two main ways in which cells may produce and maintain a state of immunity. They are macrophage activation and lymphocyte cytotoxicity. There are also several mechanisms involved in the production of a state of delayed hypersensitivity which contribute to pathology.

1. Specificity sensitized T-lymphocytes, produced in the paracortical areas of lymphoid tissues, enter the circulation and 'home' onto the site or sites containing antigen. In the case of leprosy this is predominantly the infected macrophages of the skin and nerves. Here TH (CD4) cells recognise antigen, appropriately presented by an antigen presenting cell with the appropriate HLA molecules, and driven by interleukin 2, secrete gamma interferon. This lymphokine inhibits the migration of macrophages, thus playing a part in the focalization of the lesion, and more importantly triggers the 'respiratory burst', a chain of enzymatic reactions that produces H_2O_2 which kills intracellular organisms. The capacity of macrophages to digest killed organisms is also increased (Fig. 7.3). This process will continue, and be augmented by the recruitment of more lymphocytes, so long as antigen is being presented and T-cells capable of producing and recognizing interleukin 2 are present.

2. Tc (CD8) cells respond in a similar way but they secrete lymphotoxins which destroy the antigen bearing cells. They may be responsible for caseation in tuberculosis, ulceration in cutaneous leishmaniasis and destruction of cancer and virus-infected cells. CD8 cells are prominent in leprosy lesions, but their role is poorly understood.

Lymphokines. Lymphokines are not immunoglobulins. They are mainly glycoproteins and have a very short range of action: their effect is therefore only local, in contrast to that of circulating antibody. In addition to *interleukin 2*, *gamma interferon* and *lymphotoxins*, activated lymphocytes produce several other lymphokines originally identified and known by their biological activity. These included *skin reactive factor*, which increases capillary permeability, *chemotactic factor*, which attracts macrophages, *tumour necrosis factor*, and *mitogenic factor* which causes lymphocytes that are not specifically sensititised to divide and secrete lymphokines, thus augmenting the response. The use of monoclonal antibodies has led to the identification of many lymphokines, and their reclassification (Table 7.2).

These events create the phenomena of cell mediated immunity and delayed hypersensitivity that are seen in tissues. These are:

1. Focalization and division of macrophages.

Table 7.2 Lymphokines produced by activated T-helper cells: a simplified guide. (IL1 is produced by macrophages: see text)

Designation	Target cell	Activity
IL2	B	proliferation
	T_H	proliferation, lymphokine production
	Tc NK	stimulation
IL3	stem cells	stimulation
IL4 (BCGF, MAF)	B	proliferation
	T	proliferation
	macrophages	epithelioid cell formation
IL5 (Eo-CSF)	eosinophils	differentiation
IL6	hepatocytes	production of acute phase proteins
INFγ (MAF)	B	proliferation
	NK	stimulation
	macrophages	increased microbicidal and tumoricidal activity
GMCSF	macrophages, polymorphs	stimulates
TNFα	macrophages	activates
TNF β (cachectin)	hepatocytes	inhibits protein synthesis

IL: interleukin; BCGF: B-cell growth factor; MAF: macrophage activation factor; Eo-CSF: eosinophil colony stimulating factor; GMCSF: granulocyte macrophage colony stimulating factor; TNF: tumour necrosis factor.

2. Accumulation of lymphocytes around the macrophages.
3. Alteration of macrophages into epithelioid cells, often with the formation of giant cells. Steps 1, 2 and 3 produce a tubercle, the characteristic histological picture of cell mediated immunity. This is a function of interleukin 4.
4. Increased enzymatic activity of macrophages and increased ability to phagocytose and digest organisms. This increased activity is not specific to the organism inducing the immune response.
5. Central necrosis, or ulceration of overlying skin.

When the end result of these processes is elimination of invading organisms and protection against reinfection a state of cell mediated immunity exists; when inflammation alone, cellular or delayed hypersensitivity exists.

Regulation and suppression of the immune response

Regulation

Some of the normal regulatory systems are shown in Figure 7.3. Ts cells suppress the response of TH cells to antigen and may inhibit the replication of activated B-cells. The mechanism by which they do this is not understood. Antibody regulates the immune response in several ways. IgG antibody forms complexes with antigen which inhibit B-lymphocyte proliferation. Antibody may mask antigen on presenting cells. The part of the variable region of the 'closed jaws' of the Fab part of an immunoglobulin molecule is known as an idiotype: it has a molecular configuration that is specific to an antigen. During an antigen-antibody response, these jaws are opened and idiotypes are exposed. Idiotypes are themselves antigenic and induce anti-idiotypic antibodies, thus creating an endless regulatory network. In addition to modulating antibody response, anti-idiotype antibodies, whose own variable region has the con-formation of the original antigen, suppress TH activity, presumably by competing for the antigen recognition site. A strong antigenic stimulus, for example by *M. leprae*, induces an intense polyclonal antibody response to related and unrelated antigens.

Suppression

Immune suppression may arise from overregulation, especially if part of the effector arm is inefficient, or from abnormalities in the response. A T-cell clone, or an Ir gene, may be absent. The T-cell clone may be killed by antigen induced tolerance. Free antigen may preferentially induce suppressor cells. Some antigens, even when appropriately presented, induce Ts rather than TH cells. *M. leprae* has such antigens. Failure to switch from IgM to IgG antibody production, with the persistent overproduction of IgM, may mask antigen from T-cells, or withhold the effector and regulatory roles of IgG antibody. Lymphoid tissue that is preoccupied by the presence of one antigen may respond poorly to another (antigenic competition). Such a mechanism might contribute to the partial suppression of cellular immunity which is found in some cases of LL leprosy.

Pregnancy suppresses cellular immunity, and affects the pattern of leprosy (see p. 53). Some diseases impair the immune response, including malaria, measles and malnutrition. The effect of these on a primary leprosy infection is unknown. Some drugs, the commonest of which are the corticosteroids, are immunosuppressive. This knowledge is made use of in the treatment of reactions. The effect of HIV viruses on infection with *M. leprae* is unknown. Will leprosy become an AIDS disease?

IMMUNOLOGICAL FINDINGS IN LEPROSY

The pathological and clinical characteristics of leprosy form a spectrum from LL to TT. The factor which mainly determines the place of an individual patient's disease on this spectrum is the extent to which the cell mediated immunity is expressed. In tuberculoid leprosy cellular immunity and hypersensitivity are well developed. In lepromatous leprosy they are absent; in LL induction and/or expression may be impaired. In borderline disease expression rather than induction is impaired. In addition the antibody responses at the poles differ and although this difference may not directly contribute to the patient's position on the spectrum, it does contribute to certain other aspects of the disease.

Characteristics of the immune response at the poles

Tuberculoid leprosy

1. Cellular response. The presence of cellular immunity is shown by certain characteristics of disease at this pole and by some experimental data (Fig. 7.4).

a. The essential histological characteristic is the tubercle: specialized macrophages (epithelioid cells) focalized by lymphocytes. In the central granuloma are TH cells (CD4 cells) and cells with

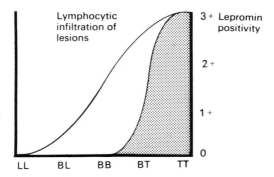

Fig. 7.4 Cell mediated immune response, as shown by lymphocytic infiltration of lesions and by lepromin positivity (shaded).

receptors for interleukin 2. In the mantle are TH cells, Ts/c (CD8 cells) and cells producing interleukin 2. HLA class II antigens are richly expressed by immunocompetent cells. These findings suggest organization into an expanding core of helper cells driven by interleukin 2, and leading to macrophage activation and bacillary destruction, and a peripheral regulatory zone of suppressor/cytotoxic cells.

b. Delayed cutaneous hypersensitivity is present and is shown by a positive lepromin test (see below).

c. Lymph nodes show well developed paracortical areas containing pyroninophilic blast cells. Intermediary sinuses contain numerous non-pyroninophilic lymphocytes. Germinal centres are poorly developed and medullary cords contain few plasma cells.

d. Lymphocytes from patients with tuberculoid leprosy, cultured in vitro in the presence of leprosy bacilli, transform into blast cells, activate macrophages and inhibit their migration. The degree of lymphocyte transformation correlates with the position of the patient's disease on the spectrum, and the intensity of inflammation of skin lesions. Special culture techniques, however, have also shown the presence of circulating, suppressive, CD8 cells.

e. Macrophages from patients with tuberculoid leprosy can be stimulated, in vitro, to digest *M. leprae* if lymphocytes from a tuberculoid patient (but not from a lepromatous patient) are added to the culture.

f. The disease tends to heal spontaneously.

2. Humoral response.

a. Antibodies to antigens of *M. leprae* can be detected in sera of

Table 7.3 Antibodies across the leprosy spectrum

Antigen	Antibody class	specificity	activity	Assay system	Patients (% +ve)				Contacts (% +ve)	
					LL	BL	BT	TT	MBL	PBL
Whole *M. leprae*		*M. leprae*		FLA-ABS[1]	100	94	82	74	18–90	
Sonicated *M. leprae*	IgG,M	mycobacteria	precipitation	GP[2]	50			10	73	33
Sonicated *M. leprae*	IgG,M	mycobacteria	precipitation	CIE[3]						
Antigen 7	IgG,M,A	mycobacteria		RIA[4]	30–80*		0–60			
Whole *M. leprae*	IgM	?		ELISA	100		0			
	IgG				100		54		10–55	
Phenolic glycolipid	IgM	*M. leprae*		ELISA or SPOT[5]	100		46			
Synthetic glycolipid	IgM	*M. leprae*		ELISA[6]	90		25			
Epitope	monoclonal	*M. leprae*		ELISA[7] or RIA	100		47			

1. Indirect immunofluorescence after absorption of sera against other mycobacterial species makes the test specific for *M. leprae*. It is useful in epidemiology. High titres indicate persistence of *M. leprae* which makes the test useful in identifying subclinical, especially pre-lepromatous cases. The test is time-consuming, laborious and subjective.

2. Gel precipitation is laborious and insensitive and cannot demonstrate *M. leprae* specific antibodies.

3. Crossed immunoelectrophoresis. Difficult test, useful experimentally to identify antigens and antibodies, but not of diagnostic or epidemiological value.

4. Radioimmunoassay enables responses to a chosen antigen to be studied. * Figures show % maximal binding to the antigen. Antibodies demonstrated in 30% of babies of leprosy patients. IgA antibodies have been shown in cord blood of infants and mucosae of adults.

5. Spot test uses antigen fixed to a card and is simpler than ELISA. Antibody titres to phenolic glycolipid reflect the bacillary load. Antibody titres disappear gradually after treatment in paucibacillary disease but persist in 50% of patients with multibacillary disease. IgM antibodies fade first.

6. Enzyme-linked immunosorbent assay is a simple test, suitable for mass use. The detection of specific IgM antibodies is potentially ideal for identifying subclinical lepromatous patients.

7. This is an inhibition assay in which the monoclonal competes with the test serum for specific epitopes. Subclinical cases of LL have high titres by this test. Monoclonals can also be used to demonstrate antigens in tissue and to *identify M. leprae* in e.g. insects.

patients with TT leprosy but at a lower frequency and titre than in LL leprosy (Table 7.3).

b. Auto-antibodies are not produced.

Lepromatous leprosy

1. Cellular response. The absence of cellular immunity is shown in the following ways:

a. There is no tubercle formation. The histological picture is that of the leproma: undifferentiated macrophages, often damaged by oedema and full of bacilli, with no surrounding lymphocytes. Live and dead bacilli are surrounded by a 'foam' of phenolic glycolipid. There is no organization of granuloma into core and mantle. TH (CD4) and especially Ts/c (CD8) cells are scattered sparsely throughout. Few cells are producing interleukin 2, about 20 times less than in a tuberculoid granuloma, but cells with receptors for interleukin 2, are as numerous. Injection of interleukin 2, or gamma interferon, into lepromatous lesions induced local upgrading with clearing of *M. leprae* from the local area.

b. The lepromin test is negative.

c. Lymph nodes show well developed germinal centres and medullary cords full of plasma cells. Paracortical areas are poorly developed and are replaced by undifferentiated and often bacilliferous macrophages. Intermediary sinuses do not contain lymphocytes.

d. Lymphocytes from patients with lepromatous leprosy do not transform in vitro into blast cells in the presence of *M. leprae*, nor do they activate macrophages or inhibit their migration, nor do they produce gamma interferon. This in vitro defect is partly reversible in a proportion of patients by the addition of interleukin 2. The number of circulating lymphocytes, capable of binding *M. leprae* to their surface, is much lower in lepromatous than tuberculoid patients.

Some, but not all investigators, using special culture techniques have shown the presence of circulating Ts cells — possibly different from those demonstrable in tuberculoid patients. When cultured with *M. leprae*, the phenolic glycolipid or the 36 kd antigen, these cells suppress the responses of HLA-D matched TH cells to antigens of *M. leprae*. Removal of Ts cells partially restores in vitro responsiveness in a proportion of LL patients. The significance of these in vitro observations, which are not universally accepted, is unclear.

e. Macrophages from lepromatous patients can be stimulated in vitro to digest *M. leprae* if lymphocytes from a tuberculoid patient (but not from a lepromatous) are added to the culture. Macrophages from lepromatous patients produce a monokine that inhibits the production of interleukin 2.

    f. The disease does not heal spontaneously.

    2. Humoral response (Fig. 7.5).

    a. Antibodies to antigens of *M. leprae* and other mycobacteria can be detected in high titre by complement fixation, precipitation, indirect haemagglutination, immunofluorescence and enzyme-linked immunosorbent assay (ELISA) see Table 7.3. Precipitins to up to 5 antigens are present in 80% of lepromatous sera. Serum levels of IgG are raised.

    b. Sera from lepromatous patients do not inhibit, in vitro, the blastogenic response to *M. leprae* of lymphocytes from tuberculoid patients. This observation implies the absence of enhancing antibodies in those sera.

    c. Many auto-antibodies are produced. They include specific antibodies such as those against thyroid, nerve, testis and gastric mucosa, and cross-reactive antibodies such as rheumatoid factor (anti-immunoglobulin), anti-DNA, cryoglobulins and cardiolipin that gives rise to false positive tests for syphilis in the Wassermann reaction.

Antibodies in leprosy do not seem to have any protective or useful role. They are unable to get at the intracellular organism. They play a role in type II reactions, but in doing so are of no benefit to the patient. It is not known whether autoimmune antibodies cause tissue damage, result from tissue damage or are a manifestation of the adjuvant activity of *M. leprae* in lymph nodes and not directly related to the clinical or pathological pattern of leprosy.

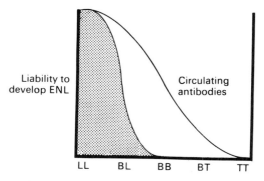

Fig. 7.5 Humoral response as shown by presence of precipitating antibodies in serum and liability to develop erythema nodosum leprosum (shaded).

Nature of immune deficiency in lepromatous leprosy

The immunological findings in leprosy indicate that there is a deficiency of cellular immunity to *M. leprae* in patients with lepromatous disease. The clone of lymphocytes which should respond is absent or unresponsive or responds abnormally. The end result is that there is inadequate production of interleukin 2, gamma interferon and other lymphokines, so that the granuloma is not organized, macrophages are not activated and are unable to digest *M. leprae*. Other features of cellular hypersensitivity are also absent. The present evidence suggests that clones of T-lymphocytes responsive to *M. leprae* exist, but that TH cells are not induced or are unable to multiply, perhaps because of failure to produce IL2 when re-stimulated by antigen. Some studies suggest that by contrast Ts cells are produced, capable of inhibiting what little TH function may exist. In addition TH cells responsive to other mycobacteria fail to respond to the cross-reactive epitopes of *M. leprae*, so that lepromatous patients fail to get this extra non-specific help. HLA-DR is expressed in lepromatous patients but the Ir gene HLA-DR3 is inherited less often than in tuberculoid patients while HLA-DQW3 is inherited more often (see p. 97). It remains possible that the defect is under genetic control. Otherwise one must postulate that the initial recognition of *M. leprae* by the patient induced tolerance (see p. 94). This defect is normally absolute and irreversible in LL.

In BB and BL, and in some patients classified as having LL, the defect is reversible after chemotherapy and antigen clearance. In vitro manipulation may also partially reverse the defect in a proportion of patients. This suggests that additional, reversible factors are suppressing cellular immunity. These may be products of *M. leprae* such as antigens with suppressive epitopes, or products of the immune response such as immune complexes, enhancing or idiotypic antibodies or overproduction of regulatory Ts cells. Suppressive factors produced by macrophages in LL may also contribute.

The severe deficiency of cellular immunity in LL is specific for *M. leprae*. There is, however, a partial generalized depression of cellular immunity in some patients with severe LL. They have a reduced number of circulating T-lymphocytes, and in vitro tests of lymphocyte function to other antigens may be slightly impaired. Their response to sensitization with some, but not all, chemical agents (e.g. dinitrochlorobenzene) is impaired, their responses to several skin test antigens are depressed, they reject grafts of homologous skin more slowly and they may be more susceptible to intercurrent disease. This depression, which tends to recover after treatment, is possibly due to disorganization of lymph node architecture and to antigenic competition.

Lepromin test

Lepromin is a crude semi-standardized preparation of bacilli from a lepromatous nodule, or an armadillo liver.

0.1 ml is injected intradermally and the site is examined after 72 hours (Fernandez reaction), and three or four weeks (Mitsuda reaction) for a palpable nodule whose diameter is measured and graded:

No nodule	Negative
1 to 2 mm	± (doubtful)
3 to 5 mm	+
over 5 mm	+ +
Ulceration	+ + +

A positive Fernandez reaction indicates the presence of delayed hypersensitivity to antigens of *M. leprae*, and is an indication of previous infection with this or a cross-reacting *Mycobacterium*. A positive Mitsuda reaction may indicate *either* that the person has previously been exposed to antigens of *M. leprae* and has developed cellular hypersensitivity *or* that he is capable of mounting a specific cell mediated response to *M. leprae*, and so is of prognostic value (see p. 212).

The test is positive in cases of TT and BT leprosy, but cannot be used for diagnosis. There is some degree of cross-reactivity with antigens of other *Mycobacteria*. Infection with *M. tuberculosis*, immunization with BCG or previous skin testing with lepromin may, but does not necessarily, induce Mitsuda positivity in a healthy person.

Leprolin and leprosin

These are soluble extracts of *M. leprae* and have been used to test for delayed hypersensitivity in epidemiological studies. The antigens are not specific and the interpretation of positive results is difficult.

FURTHER READING

Baohong J, Ouankui T, Yenlong L et al 1984 The sensitivity and specificity of fluorescent leprosy antibody absorption (FLA-ABS) test for detecting subclinical infection in leprosy. Leprosy Review 55: 327–335
Coombs R R A, Gell P G H 1986 Classification of allergic reactions responsible for clinical hypersensitivity and disease. In: Gell P G H, Coombs R A (eds) Clinical aspects of immunology. Blackwell, Oxford, pp 575–596

Godal T, Myklestad B, Samuel D R, Myrvang B 1971 Characterization of cellular immune defect in lepromatous leprosy: A specific lack of circulating *Mycobacterium leprae* — reactive lympocytes. Clinical and Experimental Immunology 9: 821–831

Hansel T T 1987 Leucocyte typing — OKCD? Lancet ii: 1382–1383

Kaplan G, Cohn Z A 1986 Regulation of cell mediated immunity in lepromatous leprosy. Leprosy Review 57 (52): 199–207

Meeker H C, Levis W R, Sersen E, Schuller Levis G, Brennan P J, Buchanan T 1986 ELISA detection of IgM antibodies against phenolic glycolipid I in the management of leprosy: a comparison between laboratories. International Journal of Leprosy 54: 530–539

Melsom R 1983 Serodiagnosis of leprosy: the past, the present and the prospects for the future. International Journal of Leprosy 51: 235–252

Modlin R L, Hofman F M, Horowitz A, Husmann L A, Gillis S, Taylor C R, Rea T H 1984 *In situ* identification of cells in human leprosy granulomas with monoclonal antibodies to interleukin 2 and its receptor. Journal of Immunology 132: 3085–3090

Nath I, Sathish M, Jayaraman T, Bhuktani L K, Sharma A K 1984 Evidence for the presence of *M. leprae* reactive T lymphocytes in patients with lepromatous leprosy. Clinical and Experimental Immunology 58: 522–530

Nelson E E, Wong L, Uyemura A, Rea T H, Modlin R L 1987 Lepromin induced suppressor cells in lepromatous leprosy. Cellular Immunology 104: 99–104

O'Garra A, Umland S, de France T, Christiansen J 1988 'B-cell factors' are pleiotropic. Immunology Today 9: 2, 45–53

Ottenhoff T H M, de Vries R R P 1987 HLA Class II immune response and suppression genes in leprosy. (Reprinted article), International Journal of Leprosy 53; 521–534

Shankar P, Agis F, Wallach D, Flagenl B, Cottenot F, Augier S, Bach M A 1986 *M. leprae* and PPD-triggered T cell lines in tuberculoid and lepromatous leprosy. Journal of Immunology 136: 4255–4263

Skinsness O K 1973 Immunopathology of leprosy. International Journal of Leprosy 41: 329–360

Turk J L, Bryceson A D M 1971 Immunological phenomena in leprosy and related diseases. Advances in Immunology 13: 209–266

8. Immunological complications: reactions

The term reaction is used to describe the appearance of symptoms and signs of acute inflammation in the lesions of a patient with leprosy.

Clinically there is swelling, redness and tenderness of skin lesions and swelling, pain and tenderness of nerves, accompanied very often by loss of function. New lesions may make their appearance. It is important to recognize and treat reactions promptly because nerve damage may be rapid and extensive. Reactions probably represent an episode of acute hypersensitivity to bacillary antigens, brought about by a disturbance of the pre-existing immunological balance. Two kinds of hypersensitivity are thought to underlie the bewildering array of clinical manifestations that may appear during reactions (Fig. 8.1).

The first (type 1) is cellular hypersensitivity and often, but not invariably, accompanies an alteration in the degree of cellular immunity exhibited by the patient, whose disease then undergoes a corresponding shift along the spectrum. It follows that reactions of this type occur in patients with borderline disease (BL, BB, BT) whose immunological status is unstable. The change in cellular immunity of the patient may be in either direction. The term *reversal* is used for an increase in immunity and a shift towards the tuberculoid pole and the term *downgrading* for a loss of immunity and a shift towards the lepromatous pole. Reversal commonly follows treatment; downgrading only occurs in a patient who is not receiving adequate treatment and is often precipitated by puberty in the male and pregnancy or parturition in the female. Despite this fundamental difference, reactions accompanying reversal and downgrading are often clinically indistinguishable and are conveniently considered together.

The second (type 2) is humoral hypersensitivity and is not associated with a shift along the spectrum. It is due to an antigen-antibody reaction with the formation of immune complexes at the site of antigen depots in various tissues and gives rise to acute inflammatory foci. It follows that this type of reaction occurs in patients at the

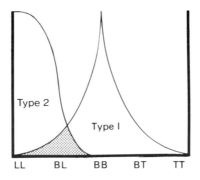

Fig. 8.1   Liability to reactions.

lepromatous end of the spectrum (LL and to a lesser extent BL) (Fig. 8.1)

A third type of reaction, the Lucio phenomenon, is a vasculitis centred upon *M. Leprae* in vascular endothelial cells and is more severe than type 2 reactions, with which it has similarities (see p. 124).

Under the Gell and Coombs classification of immunologically mediated mechanisms of tissue damage, leprosy reactions types 1 and 2, would be examples, respectively, of Type IV and Type III mechanisms.

TYPE 1 REACTIONS

Clinical features

Near the tuberculoid pole

Skin lesions become swollen and oedematous (Fig. 8.2). Erythema is often followed by desquamation and sometimes by ulceration (Fig. 8.3, Plate 5). If a facial lesion embraces the eye or nose there may be conjunctival oedema, itching and lacrimation, or nasal stuffiness. Not all the lesions are necessarily involved. In patients undergoing reversal, new lesions are unusual; but when they appear they present well defined tuberculoid characteristics with discrete and thickly infiltrated margins. Such reactions were once considered favourable as the patient's leprosy often tended to heal spontaneously, but this was at the expense of his nerves.

The nearer the patient is to the centre of the spectrum the greater is the number of lesions that become involved, and the more severe the

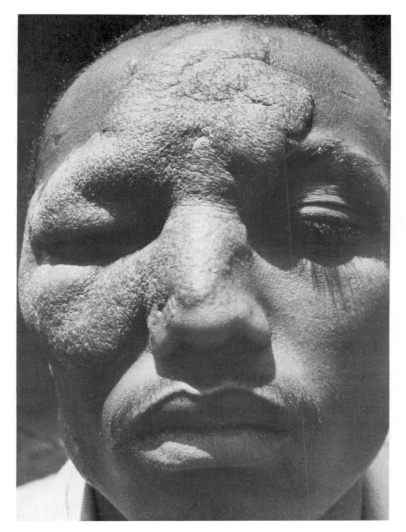

Fig. 8.2   Major tuberculoid (BT) lesion in reaction. Large, well-defined lesions of BT leprosy are often on the face and are especially prone to severe reactions. Note the gross oedema of the lesion which could ulcerate and form a scar unless an anti-inflammatory drug is used. The conjunctiva of the right eye was oedematous and uncomfortable.

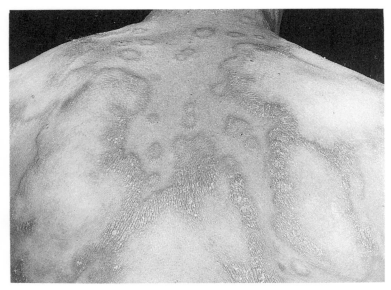

Fig. 8.3 Type 1 reaction in borderline tuberculoid leprosy, upgrading from BL, in an Anglo-Indian during treatment. The lesions are inflamed, as shown by desquamation, and in a pale skin are erythematous. During the reaction several new well defined plaques have appeared. Compare these lesions with those of BB leprosy (Fig. 4.14) and those seen in downgrading (Fig. 4.25).

changes. During downgrading many new lesions may appear and these will tend not to show the marginal definition of the pre-existing lesions (Figs 4.25, 4.26 Plate 5). After each reaction the lesions assume more borderline characteristics. Tenosynovitis, especially of the extensor tendons over the back of the wrist, may develop during reactions in borderline leprosy (Fig. 8.4).

Nerves. The few nerves that are affected will become rapidly swollen, extremely painful and tender. Paraesthesiae or pain in their sensory distribution is common. Loss of motor function develops rapidly. This may become permanent if not treated quickly. Pure neural leprosy (see p. 42) may present in this way. Sudden paralysis due to radial, ulnar or lateral popliteal neuritis carries a better prognosis than that due to facial nerve damage. Systemic illness is minimal, often confined to oedema of the limbs or face.

In the centre of the spectrum

Reactions in patients with BB leprosy may be extremely severe, possibly because they are associated with the greatest degree of shift.

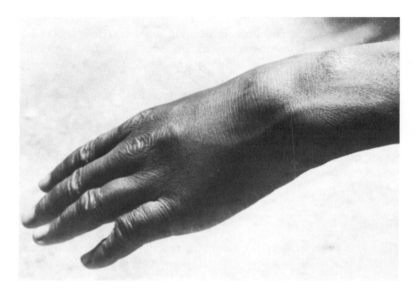

Fig. 8.4 Type 1 reaction in borderline leprosy. Leprous infiltration of the soft tissues of the hand can be the site of reactional inflammation. In this case there is tenosynovitis shown by swelling over the dorsum of the wrist, and oedema of the fingers. Early damage to the ulnar nerve is shown by slight flexion and abduction of the little finger.

Skin lesions become rapidly swollen, erythematous and oedematous. Pain in the lesions and tenderness are severe. Numerous new lesions may appear.

Nerves. Many nerves are involved, and become swollen, painful and tender. Widespread nerve damage with extensive paresis follows. The patient is immobilized by pain and weakness.

Systemic illness is more common, with weakness, malaise and generalized oedema, especially of the hands, feet and face.

Near the lepromatous pole

Type 1 reactions, appearing for the first time in BL leprosy, usually represent upgrading, and are commonest in patients who show signs of having recently downgraded and are now starting to receive treatment. Such reactions may last for many months and demand careful management.

Skin lesions increase rapidly in size and definition. They become red, shiny and tense. New lesions appear and the whole skin may become infiltrated.

Nerves. Although most of the peripheral nerves are likely to be involved, the degree of cellular infiltration is not as great at this end of the spectrum and there is less likelihood of rapidly progressive paralysis. Nevertheless, in some patients individual nerves may be greatly enlarged, painful and damaged.

Systemic illness. Fever, malaise and prostration can be severe with daily temperature spikes, and oedema.

Untreated patients may also downgrade and suffer the effects of bacillary invasion of the mucosa of the upper respiratory tract, eye, testes and phalanges. As cellular hypersensitivity is suppressed, type 2 reactions may take over and the clinical picture becomes complicated (see p. 122).

Histology

Histologically reactions accompanying reversal and downgrading are usually distinguishable, especially if there has been a previous biopsy for comparison.

Reversal is characterized by oedema and an increase in lymphocytic infiltration and of the volume of the lesion. Macrophage differentiation towards epithelioid cells increases and giant cells take on the appearance of Langhans' cells. The number of bacilli decreases and the morphological index falls. Occasionally there is necrosis within the granuloma. Healing is accompanied by fibrosis.

Downgrading is characterized by loss of focalization and of tubercle formation. The number of lymphocytes in the lesion diminishes and epithelioid cells de-differentiate towards more simple histiocytes and may show intracellular oedema. These changes are followed by an increase of bacillary multiplication and a rising morphological index. Extracellular oedema is also present. The granuloma spreads and there is no accompanying fibrosis.

Immunology

Reactions during reversal may happen spontaneously, especially in subpolar BT leprosy, but more usually follow reduction in bacillary load as a result of treatment. The gain in cellular immunity results in an improved prognosis, with more rapid progress towards healing and decreasing liability to relapse. The Bacterial Index falls. If the patient's disease shifts from BL or BB to BT, the lepromin test will become positive.

Reactions during downgrading happen spontaneously in untreated patients and in patients whose treatment has been interrupted for any reason. The loss of CMI may lead to a rapid downhill course. The Bacterial Index rises. If the patient's disease shifts from the BT part of the spectrum, the lepromin test will become negative.

Sequential in vitro studies in untreated Indian patients presenting in reaction, showed that of those with BT leprosy roughly half were upgrading and half downgrading, while all of those with BL leprosy were upgrading.

The cause of the acute inflammation which is the essential feature of type 1 reactions is a sudden increase in cellular hypersensitivity, which is demonstrated by a sudden increase in lymphocyte transformation (see p. 103). Reactions accompanying upgrading show increased organisation into core and mantle with an influx of CD8 cells in the mantle (p. 106). Studies in vitro have suggested that hypersensitivity is directed mainly against cytoplasmic antigens during reactions in nerves, and mainly against surface antigens during reactions in skin. In reactions accompanying reversal, hypersensitivity increases with immunity, possibly in response to antigens released from killed bacilli. In reactions without a shift along the spectrum, episodes of hypersensitivity occur without any change in immunity. These two situations may be compared with the positive responses to Mantoux tests (episodes of hypersensitivity) in patients with tuberculosis whose disease is getting better (reversal) or staying the same (no shift). Reactions seen during downgrading probably represent a relative increase in cellular hypersensitivity elicited by the increased secretion of antigens by multiplying bacilli, which itself represents a decrease in immunity (like a Mantoux test with a very large dose of tuberculin in a patient whose tuberculosis is getting worse: downgrading). It is also possible that the generalized oedema and fever which sometimes accompanies reactions may correspond in some way to the Koch phenomenon in tuberculosis: a situation in which the systemic injection of a large dose of tuberculin induces oedema, fever and malaise.

TYPE 2 REACTIONS

Clinical features

Type 2 reactions, which complicate LL and BL leprosy, may arise spontaneously but are commonest in patients who have had enough treatment to reduce the morphological index to under 5%. Over half the number of patients under treatment for LL will suffer type 2 reactions at some time and about one-quarter of those with BL. Reactions are particularly common during pregnancy and lactation. Attacks are frequently prolonged or recurrent.

The reaction is characterized by erythema nodosum leprosum (ENL), the appearance in the skin of painful red nodules, which may be superficial or deep in the dermis (Fig. 8.5, 8.6). They are dome shaped with ill-defined margins, shiny and tender. They may ulcerate, discharging thick yellow pus which contains polymorphs and degenerate acid-fast bacilli, but is sterile on culture. Lesions are commonest on the face and extensor surfaces of the limbs, but may also be seen elsewhere. Lesions last for a few days and may be succeeded by crops of new ones. As they fade they become purplish in colour, difficult to see on dark skins, and the surrounding skin feels thickened. Chronic ENL shows as a brawny induration most frequently over the extensor surfaces of thighs, calves and forearms.

In addition any or several of the following manifestations may appear: (iridocyclitis (see p. 158), orchitis, dactylitis, tender enlargement of all peripheral nerves and tender lymphadenopathy. Less commonly, muscles may be tender and joints may be painful or even

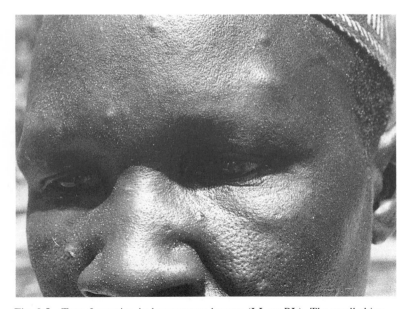

Fig. 8.5 Type 2 reaction in lepromatous leprosy (LL or BL). The small shiny nodules on the forehead are typical of erythema nodosum leprosum which characterizes mild type 2 reactions. The lesions were painful and in lighter skins would be erythematous. Note also the oedema of the left cheek.

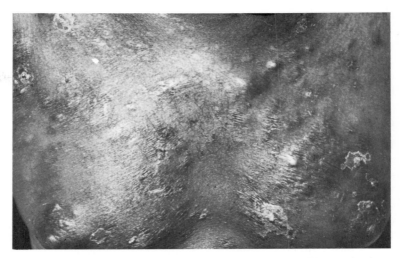

Fig. 8.6 Type 2 reaction in lepromatous leprosy (LL or BL). The reaction here is worse than in Figure 8.5. There is inflammation of large areas of skin; several discrete lesions are pustular and some of them have broken down. Compare this picture of ENL with that of BL leprosy in Figure 4.24. Note also the gynaecomastia.

swollen, and there may be epistaxis and proteinuria. Fever, headache, insomnia due to pain and depression can be troublesome. Occasionally iridocyclitis may be the only sign of reaction, or even of leprosy. Type 2 reactions are not usually of such serious significance as type 1 reactions, because they are often confined to skin, and nerve damage is seldom as rapid, but they are often more prolonged. The presence of neuritis or iridocyclitis, however, calls for vigorous anti-inflammatory treatment. In severe cases the accompanying systemic illness may be extremely debilitating.

Histology

In the majority of cases of mild ENL, the focus of inflammation is away from the major skin lesions, and often deep in the dermis. There are, however, usually a few bacilli at the centre of the reaction site. The bacilli are often fragmented or granular, and even after they cannot be shown by carbol-fuchsin, their ghosts can be shown by electron microscopy, and antigens by immunofluorescence, bound to macrophages and connective tissue. Mild lesions consist of collections of polymorphs, oedema and cellular disintegration. Vasculitis or vascular necrosis with haemorrhage is present in some but not all lesions. Severe ENL is more often associated with larger bacillary deposits. Polymorph infiltration is intense and may extend through large areas of the dermis, and there may be much oedema. Necrosis and ulceration may follow. A similar polymorph infiltration is found in the ciliary body, nerves, muscle and lymph nodes when they are involved.

Immunology

Patients with lepromatous leprosy have high titres of precipitating antibody to antigens of *M. leprae*. For most of the time these do not seem to play any role in the pathology of the disease. On occasion, however, the relative concentrations of antigen and precipitating antibody would seem to be appropriate for the formation of immune complexes which are then deposited in the tissues. Complement is fixed to the deposited complex, and polymorphonuclear leucotactic factor is released. Polymorphs accumulate, phagocytose the complexes and release proteolytic enzymes which produce inflammation and necrosis of tissue. The formation of complexes can take place either in the tissues, where there is a concentration gradient of antigen as it diffuses away from a clump of degenerating bacilli, or in the circulation. During episodes of ENL circulating complexes containing complement (Clq), IgG and IgM have been demonstrated. In the former situation foci of inflammation will develop in or near pre-existing lesions; and if complexes have been deposited in the wall of a blood vessel, which represents the origin of the antibody gradient, there will be vasculitis. In the latter situation circulating immune complexes will be formed and deposited at sites distant from the bacilliferous lesions. This mechanism may account for the eruption of erythematous nodules in the skin at sites apparently previously unaffected, and for nephritis, and may contribute to the genesis of arthralgia and neuritis, which are features also of other circulating immune complex disease, such as serum sickness.

During type 2 reactions there is an increase in the ratio of CD4 to CD8 lymphocytes and a decrease in the number of CD8. This suggests that a cellular immune mechanism in some way regulates expression of inflammation due to immune complexes; however, there is no shift in position of the patient's disease along the immunological spectrum, no alteration of lepromin negativity and no change in the prognosis.

LUCIO PHENOMENON

This occurs exclusively in patients with Lucio leprosy (see p. 40),

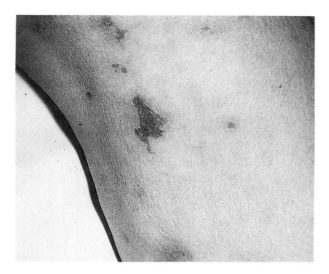

Fig. 8.7   Early Lucio phenomenon: a typical haemorrhagic infarct approximately 36 hours old. It will break down and form a deep ulcer. A small halo of erythema surrounds the haemorrhagic area. The serrated irregular margins are typical.

often before treatment has been started. Small pink lesions appear on the skin, usually on a limb. They are ill-defined, painful and just palpable, and commonly triangular or irregular in shape (Fig. 8.7). After a few days they turn dark, crust and heal. Larger lesions are more inflamed, and develop overlying bullae that burst, leaving large painful ulcers that heal slowly with scarring.

Histology shows ischaemic epidermal necrosis with necrosis of superficial blood vessels and oedema and endothelial proliferation of deeper vessels. Although there is no polymorphonuclear infiltrate, as in ENL, immunofluorescent staining shows deposits of immuno-globulin and complement in the walls of the vessels, and abundant acid-fast bacilli in the endothelial cells. All patients have high titres of circulating immune complexes and cryoglobulins.

FURTHER READING

Bjune G 1983 Reactions in leprosy. Leprosy Review (special issue): 61S–67S
Bjune G, Barnetson R StC, Ridley D S, Kronvall G. 1976 Lymphocyte transformation test in leprosy; correlation of the response with inflammation of lesions. Clinical and Experimental Immunology 25: 85–94

Godal T, Myrvang B, Samuel D R, Ross W F, Løfgren M 1973 Mechanisms of 'reactions' in borderline tuberculoid leprosy. Acta Pathologica et Microbiologica Scandanavica (Sect A. Suppl.) 236: 45–53

Loal S, Misra R S, Nath I 1987 Heterogeneity in T cell functions related to background leprosy type. Type I reactions in leprosy. International Journal of Leprosy 55: 481–493

Petit J H S, Waters M F R 1967 The etiology of erythema nodosum leprosum. International Journal of Leprosy 35: 1–10

Rea T H, Ridley D S 1979 Lucio's phenomenon: a comparative histologic study. International Journal of Leprosy 47: 161–166

Ridley D S 1969 Reactions in leprosy. Leprosy Review 40: 77–81

9. Management of reactions

Untreated leprosy progresses insidiously and nerves are damaged over months or years, but during reactions acute neuritis may cripple overnight and acute iridocyclitis may lead rapidly to blindness. Inflamed skin lesions and nerves can be extremely painful. The four principles in the management of reactions are:

1. Control acute neuritis in order to prevent anaesthesia, paralysis and contracture.
2. Halt eye damage and prevent blindness.
3. Control pain.
4. Kill the bacilli and prevent extension of disease.

These principles apply regardless of the type of reaction. Although there may be differences in the management of a patient in reaction depending on type, it is the severity of the reaction that usually determines the nature of the management.

Reactions, especially type 2, may be precipitated by vaccination, intercurrent illness, hormonal disturbances such as occur during pregnancy, or even psychosocial factors. If these cannot be anticipated and prevented, they should be looked for and treated. When the patient starts treatment he should be warned that a reaction may take place. The patient must be reassured that his symptoms do not indicate a deterioration of disease, perhaps even the contrary, and that his distress can be relieved, if he seeks help promptly.

It is no longer permissible to consider that anaesthesia, paralysis and contracture are inevitable consequences of leprosy. Early diagnosis and treatment and energetic management of reactional states should prevent the development of all disabilities. A practical approach to management involves four measures.

Anti-inflammatory therapy

Mild reactions

These may be either type 1 reactions when the absence of pain and tenderness in nerves suggests that they are not in danger and the skin is not so severely inflamed that it is likely to ulcerate, or type 2 reactions confined to minor skin lesions with little systemic disturbances.

Aspirin is still the best and cheapest drug for controlling moderate degrees of pain and inflammation: 600 mg to 1200 mg are given 4 hourly, 4 to 6 times daily.

Chloroquine. The anti-inflammatory action of antimalarial drugs, of which chloroquine is the best and most readily available, is effective in controlling mild reactions: 150 mg chloroquine base is given up to 3 times daily. Toxic symptoms of prolonged chloroquine administration include rashes, especially photo-sensitization, pruritis, gastrointestinal disturbances, visual disturbances and tinnitus.

The combination of aspirin and chloroquine is often better than either alone. The dosage is reduced slowly as signs and symptoms are controlled.

Antimonials. The anti-inflammatory action of antimony may be of some benefit in controlling mild reactions. It is particularly useful in relieving pains in bones and joints in type 2 reactions. Toxic effects of antimonials include rashes, joint pains, bradycardia, hypotension and electrocardiographic changes. Organic trivalent antimonials are much less toxic than the inorganic compounds and are preferable. Stibophen contains 8.5 mg antimony per ml: 2 to 3 ml are given intramuscularly on alternate days, not exceeding a total dose of 30 ml.

Thalidomide. The anti-inflammatory effect of this drug is of use only in controlling the manifestations of type 2 reactions, including neuritis and iridocyclitis. It may be used for all but the most severe cases, and is often helpful in weaning patients off corticosteroids. It is given in a dose of 400 mg daily until the reaction is controlled, and then reduced gradually to 50 mg daily. The drug must *never* be given to pre-menopausal women because of its disastrous teratogenic effects; for which reason it is not generally available. It causes drowsiness and is best given at night. Thalidomide has been reported to cause peripheral neuritis, but this has not proved a problem in leprosy patients, even when treated for many months.

Severe reactions

Reactions considered severe are those in which:

a. Paralysis or anaesthesia threatens to follow neuritis. This is most common in type 1 reactions in BT and BB leprosy, but may occur in type 2 reactions as well.

b. Skin ulceration threatens. This may occasionally follow severe type 1 reactions, but is commonest in ENL and is often accompanied by iritis, orchitis, arthritis, dactylitis, fever and prostration.

c. Iridocyclitis or orchitis develop independently.

These conditions are medical emergencies and anti-inflammatory treatment must be undertaken energetically if disability is to be avoided. The management of iridocyclitis is given in detail on page 158.

Corticosteroids. In the case of neuritis the most rapid control is essential. In type 1 reactions prednisone or prednisolone is started in a single daily dose of 40–80 mg, according to severity. The higher dose should be reduced to 40 mg after a few days. Thereafter the dose is reduced by 5–10 mg every two to four weeks, according to response, ending with 10 mg on alternate days for at least two weeks. Response is measured by careful testing of nerve function (see p. 136). Patients with BT leprosy in reaction commonly need corticosteroids for 2–6 months, while those with BL in reaction may need them for up to nine months. For field use, a fixed regimen of 40 mg daily reducing by 5 mg every two weeks has proved safe and helpful. Cortisone or hydrocortisone are as good as prednisone; the dose is five times higher.

If a patient with type 1 reaction has been treated with dapsone plus corticosteroids, and after a period of a few weeks corticosteroids are still required at unacceptably high dosage, dapsone should be replaced by clofazimine.

In type 2 reactions nerve damage does not threaten quite so quickly as in type 1 reactions, and thalidomide is the drug of choice. If it is unavailable, or contra-indicated, prednisone should be started in a dose of 20–40 mg per day and the dose adjusted according to response. Although this lower dosage may succeed in controlling ENL the condition sometimes becomes chronic and it may be harder to wean the patient off steroids than with type 1 reactions. In this situation, the addition or increased dose of clofazimine makes it possible to withdraw steroids (see below). Occasionally thalidomide alone fails to control a type 2 reaction adequately. In this case a small additional dose of prednisone may suffice.

It must be remembered that corticosteroids suppress immune responses and thereby encourage bacillary multiplication. It is therefore doubly necessary to continue antileprosy therapy while corticosteroids are given or restart dapsone or clofazimine monotherapy if the course of triple therapy has already been completed. Other side effects of steroids include salt and water retention, the development of Cushing's syndrome with osteoporosis, diabetes, muscle wasting and the activation of peptic ulcer. Tuberculosis, strongyloidiasis and amoebiasis may flare up in patients on long-term corticosteroids treatment. When possible a chest radiograph and faecal examination should be performed.

Clofazimine. The use of clofazimine is indicated for reactions in patients who cannot be weaned off corticosteroids or who are troubled by continuous ENL and thalidomide cannot be used. Standard treatment with dapsone and rifampicin is normally continued. If the ENL has started after antileprosy chemotherapy has been stopped, no other antileprotics are needed. Clofazimine may temporarily aggravate reactions and is started under cover of an increased dose of steroids, which are then gradually withdrawn. To obtain an anti-inflammatory effect a higher dosage needs to be given than to get an antibacterial effect. Initially 300 mg is given daily in divided doses, for 2 weeks, reducing to 200 mg daily for a month or two, and then to 100 mg daily according to response. Toxic effects are given on page 84. Patients debilitated by prolonged reactions do not object to the discolouration when they are relieved of their pain and misery.

Analgesic therapy

Drugs

In mild reactions analgesics are synonymous with anti-inflammatory drugs. In severe reactions aspirin should be given in addition to corticosteroids if pain is inadequately controlled. This applies especially to chronic ENL. Where anxiety lowers the threshold to pain and insomnia is a problem chlorpromazine may be given, 25 to 50 mg up to thrice daily and at night. Opiates are rarely needed and are normally avoided because of the danger of addiction. Persisting pain is an indication for increased dosage of corticosteroid or clofazimine, or for surgery.

Intraneural injections

Intraneural injections of lignocaine and prednisone can relieve the pain of acute neuritis, but are liable to damage the nerve and increase scarring, and should be avoided. Adequate doses of systemic steroids are equally effective, and are to be preferred since they relieve infiltration in all the nerves and not just those of which the patient complains most.

Surgery

If a nerve abscess develops it may aspirated through a wide bore needle. If this fails the nerve may be exposed and the abscess incised along the axis of the nerve. Small abscesses usually resolve spontaneously.

During episodes of neuritis there is an increased volume of fluid in the nerve, the epineurium becomes thickened and the surrounding tissue swollen. These events increase intraneural pressure, especially at natural sites of constriction. If adequate corticosteroid therapy does not relieve pain or lead to a rapid improvement in nerve function, surgery may be considered. *Neurolysis* relieves the nerve from its surrounding constrictions and *epineurotomy* slits the nerve sheath, releasing internal pressure. Carried out within 10 days of the onset of reaction, by an experienced surgeon, the short- and long-term results are often good.

Nerves should *never* be stripped if there is any possibility of function remaining or returning, as this destroys blood supply, increases oedema and leads to scarring and worse damage. A nerve that has been totally functionless for many months may be slit down its length or completely excised for the relief of intractable pain.

Splinting and exercise

In severe reactions immobilization of affected limbs is helpful to relieve pain. Properly splinted limbs assist a hand or foot to survive even a severe combined type 1 and type 2 reaction and emerge with useful function. Unsplinted limbs develop contractures especially during a combined reaction in which there may be temporary paralysis and acute arthritis. The joints become stiff in the clawed position, and the hand remains disabled despite return of intrinsic muscle function. Joints should be splinted in the position of function. Splints are most conveniently made of plaster slabs or hard Plastazote®, padded with plenty of cotton wool and secured with bandages. The splint should be left in position 24 hours a day until the inflammation begins to subside, being removed only for exercise. At first gentle passive exercises are carried out daily. Active exercises are gradually introduced until complete function is restored (see also p. 172).

Antibacterial therapy

Inasmuch as leprosy is due to *M. leprae*, antibacterial therapy must be continued as long as the infection is present. This principle is especially important in the management of patients on corticosteroids and is increasingly important the nearer the patient is to the lepromatous end of the spectrum. Careful studies have shown that altering the dose of dapsone, of stopping it or restarting it, does not affect the incidence of type 2 reactions and only marginally affects their severity. Nor does rifampicin precipitate type 2 reactions.

The possible role of dapsone or rifampicin in the genesis of type 1 reactions is not completely settled (see p. 80, 121), but three points may be made about type 1 reaction:

1. In patients who present for the first time with tender nerves, clofazimine may be less likely to aggravate the situation than dapsone and rifampicin.

2. Some patients with borderline disease go into severe reaction within a few weeks after starting dapsone. A change to clofazimine may allow corticosteroids to be withdrawn sooner.

3. Whatever antileprotic drug is used during reaction it must be maintained in the usual dosage.

In type 2 reactions when ulceration of the mucosa of the upper respiratory tract occurs, streptomycin is indicated additionally (see p. 83).

Lucio's phenomenon

Chemotherapy with a regimen that contains rifampicin is the most important measure, and usually brings the phenomenon under rapid control in patients who have not yet begun treatment. Otherwise steroids should be given as for type 2 reactions. Thalidomide and clofazimine are not effective.

FURTHER READING

Becx-Bleumink M T 1989 Manual for field treatment of leprosy reactions, 2nd edn. ALERT, Addis Ababa.
Kiran K U, Stanley J A, Pearson J M H 1985 The outpatient treatment of nerve damage in patients with borderline leprosy using a semi-standardised steroid regimen. Leprosy Review 56: 127–134
Naafs B 1983 Leprosy reactions and their management, differential diagnosis with relapse. Health Cooperation Papers 1/1983: 73–76, 193
Naafs B, Pearson J M H, Wheate H W 1979 Reversal reaction: the prevention of permanent nerve damage. Comparison of short and long term steroid treatment. International Journal of Leprosy 47: 7–12
Ross W F, Pearson J M H 1975 The recognition and management of nerve damage under field conditions. Leprosy Review 46: 231–234
Waters M F R 1971 An internally controlled double blind trial of thalidomide in severe erythema nodosum leprosum. Leprosy Review 42: 26–42
Waters M F R 1974 Treatment of reactions in leprosy. Leprosy Review 45: 337–341

10. Complications due to nerve damage

Infection of peripheral nerves is an integral part of leprosy but permanent nerve damage is not an inevitable sequel of infection. Measures to prevent or reduce the reactional phases of leprosy can to a great extent minimize the amount of nerve damage. To halt and to reverse nerve pathology is of far more importance than to treat the complications occurring after irreversible changes have taken place. *Prevention of nerve damage needs to be constantly stressed as the single most important aspect of leprosy management, and one that is often neglected* (see Ch. 9).

There is a consistent pattern of nerve involvement in leprosy. Nerves are most severely affected where they lie superficially, just under the skin. In early lepromatous leprosy it is the fine terminal twigs of sensory and autonomic fibres in the skin that are affected; in tuberculoid leprosy it is major peripheral nerves at the 'sites of predilection'. It is postulated that the most likely reasons for these sites are:

1. *Temperature.* The nerves are superficial and therefore cooler. The preference of *M. leprae* for temperatures lower than body temperature supports this suggestion.

2. *Trauma* may be a factor because of the more vulnerable position of the nerves in these sites.

3. *Movement.* Damage is accentuated by constant tugging on the nerves and is usually just proximal to a joint, where there may be a tunnel through which the nerve passes, or some other form of potential constriction.

The three physiological functions of nerves, sensory, motor and autonomic, may be equally involved but usually the sensory component is the earliest and the most severely affected. Autonomic involvement seems not to be closely correlated with the other components, although with severe anaesthesia there is almost inevitably loss of sweating and vasomotor dysfunction. Frequently there is

severe and extensive sensory loss, but little or no motor weakness; and
rarely there is motor impairment with no sensory loss. Most commonly, however, there is a combination of variable degrees of
impairment of all components.

Sites of predilection of nerve involvement, and resulting disability

Ulnar nerve — just proximal to the olecranon groove. Sensation is
lost over the ulnar half of the hand. Autonomic damage causes
cyanosis and dryness. There is paresis or paralysis of the interossei and
the two medial lumbrical muscles and the muscles of the hypothenar
eminence. Atrophy follows. The little finger lies slightly abducted and
cannot be opposed, the hypothenar eminence is flattened, and there is
guttering of interosseous spaces. The ring and little fingers are flexed
at the proximal interphalangeal joints and extended at the metacarpophalangeal joints. This pattern is called ulnar or minimal claw
(Fig. 10.1). Rarely, the ulnar nerve is more extensively damaged and
there is weakness of deep flexors of the little and ring fingers.

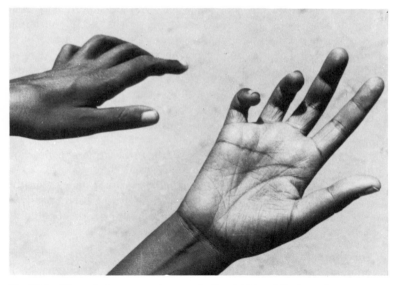

Fig. 10.1   Bilateral ulnar nerve damage. In the right hand the hypothenar
eminence is flattened and the little and ring fingers are flexed at the proximal
interphalangeal joints. The left hand shows guttering of dorsal interosseous spaces
and hyperextension at the metacarpophalangeal joints of the little and ring
fingers.

Median nerve. This is rarely involved on its own and is usually associated with ulnar nerve damage. It may be affected at two sites:

1. *Low* — just proximal to the carpal tunnel. Sensory and autonomic loss is over the lateral half of the hand. There is weakness or paralysis of muscles of the thenar eminence (opponens pollicis, abductor pollicis brevis, flexor pollicis brevis), and the two lateral lumbricals. The hand lies flat and the thumb lies in the plane of the hand. The thumb cannot be abducted or opposed, but flexion is intact. The thenar eminence is flat. The thumb, index and middle fingers are flexed at the proximal interphalangeal joints and hyperextended at the metacarpophalangeal joints (Fig. 10.2). Added to the deformity of ulnar paresis, this completes the picture of complete claw. Claw hand is at first mobile and if exercised daily can retain useful function. Neglected, contractures develop and the hand becomes fixed and function difficult to improve.

2. *High* — proximal to the bend of the elbow. This is less common. It does not increase loss of sensation, but causes loss of flexion of the index and middle fingers, and of flexion and opposition of the thumb and may weaken flexion at the wrist, and pronation.

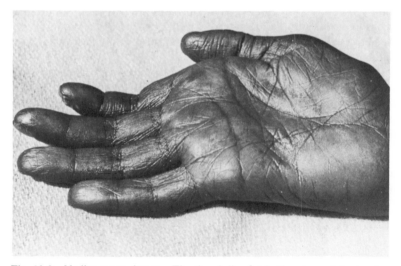

Fig. 10.2 Median nerve damage. The thumb lies flat in the plane of the hand; the thenar muscles are so wasted that the thenar eminence is concave. The thumb is flexed at the interphalangeal joint and the index and to a lesser extent middle fingers are flexed at the proximal interphalangeal joints and hyperextended at the metacarpophalangeal joints. There is also evidence of ulnar nerve damage (Fig. 8.4). The atrophic skin is a sign of autonomic nerve damage.

Radial nerve — where it winds round the humerus beneath the deltoid insertion. It is rarely involved. Sensory loss is confined to a small area proximal to the index finger on the dorsum of the hand. But motor loss is severe producing extensor and supinator paralysis with a severely disabling 'wrist drop'.

Common peroneal nerve — proximal to where the nerve passes around the neck of the fibula and extending up into the popliteal fossa. Damage to this nerve causes anaesthesia of the lateral side of the leg and the dorsum of the foot. The motor deficit is in the peroneal muscles and the dorsiflexors of the foot. The earliest sign is difficulty in dorsiflexion or eversion against pressure. The full picture is that of foot drop with a high-stepping gait.

Posterior tibial nerve — proximal to where it passes around the medial malleolus. Damage results in anaesthesia of the sole of the foot, and paralysis of the intrinsic musculature of the foot, leading to clawing of the toes, and collapse of arches. Damage to this nerve is the commonest and most important predisposing cause of injury to the feet in leprosy.

Facial nerve. (See also Ch. 11.)

1. The temporal and zygomatic branches are involved most commonly as they cross the zygoma, probably due to their superficial position at this site. Damage results in lagophthalmos, or inability to close the eyes, which in its early stage is most easily seen when the patient tries to do this gently (Fig. 4.20).

2. Paralysis of the buccal, mandibular and cervical branches is uncommon and is usually associated with involvement of the upper branches. This pattern distinguishes facial palsy in leprosy from Bell's palsy. When these branches are involved, there is loss of facial expression and inability to close the lips.

Trigeminal nerve. The pathology is probably in fine nerve endings and causes anaesthesia of the face and, most importantly, of the cornea and conjunctiva.

Tests to measure nerve function

For the purpose of diagnosis, it is adequate to perform a simple examination for anaesthesia, weakness and loss of autonomic function (see p. 58). Before treatment is begun a more detailed assessment of nerve damage is useful to provide a semi-quantitative measure of nerve damage. This is particularly important when nerve damage is recent, or threatened because of a reaction, and anti-inflammatory drugs are to be used. Periodic re-measurement provides an objective guide to management.

Sensory loss may be measured with the aid of a set of graded nylon bristles, that bend to known pressures. Motor loss is most simply measured by grading the strength of *single* muscles on the following scale:

5. Full strength
4. Slight weakness
3. Counteracts gravity
2. Cannot counteract gravity
1. Flicker of movement
0. No movement

The tests, though simple, are time-consuming and are best carried out by a trained physiotherapist.

Where facilities permit, electrophysiological tests of nerve function should be performed: nerve conduction velocity and electromyography. These tests provide quantitative measurement of individual nerve and muscle function.

Characteristics of nerve damage on the spectrum of disease

In tuberculoid leprosy nerve involvement begins early and progresses rapidly. It is due to the infiltration of the nerve by tuberculoid granuloma and to reactional oedema. The number of nerves involved is restricted, and can be compared to the few lesions of the skin seen in tuberculoid disease. At an early stage the damage can be reversed relatively easily.

In lepromatous leprosy nerve damage is widespread, but progresses much more slowly. After several years, however, there will be damage to sensory nerve endings in the cooler parts of the body such as the dorsum of the forearms, hands and feet, the ears and nose, and these parts become anaesthetic. Loss of sensation is not initially related to involvement of peripheral nerve trunks, which follows later when diffuse and extensive fibrosis replaces nerve axons, producing a pattern of anaesthesia and paralysis similar to that seen in tuberculoid leprosy, but symmetrically.

Patients with borderline leprosy have the most extensive large nerve involvement, and their liability to reactions predisposes them to the most severe damage, often with bilateral paralysis. These patients are the most difficult of all to manage.

Mechanisms causing disability

Damage to the three physiological components of nerves is followed by *anaesthesia, dryness of the skin,* and *muscular paralysis.* These three primary factors underlie deformity and disability of the hands and feet in patients with leprosy because they predispose the affected limbs to *misuse. Ulceration, scar formation* and *secondary infection* ensue, and create a vicious cycle of events which causes loss of deep tissue and results in severe disability. A further cause of damage in lepromatous patients is that due directly to *invasion of tissues by M. leprae.*

These eight causes of disability are considered in detail. Their interaction is summarised in Figure 10.3.

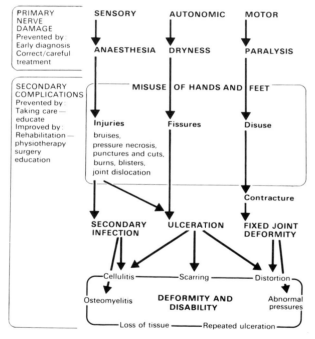

Fig. 10.3 The pathogenesis of disability following nerve damage in leprosy.

1. Anaesthesia

Anaesthesia is the most devastating complication of leprosy and by far the most important cause of disability. It greatly increases the risk of disability following motor and autonomic nerve damage, and is the main factor predisposing to secondary complications.

The how, when, where and why we touch has important psychological and behavioural functions as well as informational and protective functions. In addition to the physical injuries discussed on page 142, patients with anaesthesia suffer psychologically and socially. They feel confused, defenceless against injury, cut off from friends, afraid and even helpless. They become clumsy, have difficulty in handling things and cannot do fine work. About 50% give up some activity, such as sewing or gardening or sport, and a sense of social separation is established even before physical disability develops.

There are rare individuals with congenital absence of pain perception fibres. In the course of 15 to 30 years they develop disabilities of the hands and feet like those of people who have leprosy. The mechanism is simply lack of recognition of pain and, therefore, neglect of trauma that leads to infection of the hands and feet.

One major problem of the person who has no sensation in his limbs is to identify 'self' with 'body'. In a person with normal pain 'self' and 'body' co-exist. But a person with anaesthetic limbs considers that his 'self' does not completely fill the space of the 'body' in which his 'self' resides, and as a consequence he damages that part of the body which extends beyond the limits of 'self'. Occasionally a patient with anaesthesia of an arm will reject that arm as not part of himself, so that, even though it can function to a greater or lesser extent, he will not use it at all, and may not even put it in the sleeve of his clothes. When someone else shows interest in that limb, and begins to care for it, for example by physiotherapy, the patient will use it again and function improves.

Paul Brand, who pioneered surgical methods for the rehabilitation of leprosy patients, has said that if he had but one gift to give his patients it would be the ability to perceive pain.

2. Dryness of the skin

Damage to sympathetic nerve fibres impairs sweating and the skin becomes dry, inflexible and brittle; it fissures easily, thus starting a cycle of ulceration and scarring (Fig. 10.4). This process is most important around the margins of the sole of the foot where every step, especially of an anaesthetic foot, prevents the fissure from healing. Damage to vascular innervation in the skin and subcutaneous tissues is followed by loss of vascular tone and stasis of capillary blood. Heat may not be dissipated properly and tissues may be more readily burned. Vascular contractility is diminished and injury may more easily cause a haematoma. Oxygenation is impaired and tissues may heal less rapidly.

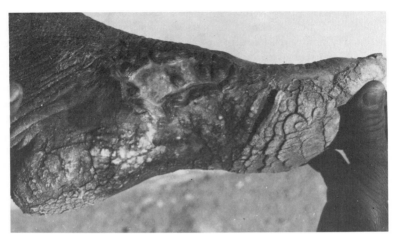

Fig. 10.4   Fissures. Autonomic nerve damage has caused the skin to become dry, and allowed fissures to form. Anaesthesia has allowed the patient to continue walking, which has deepened several fissures and, in one area, produced an extensive superficial ulcer.

3. Muscular paralysis

Paralysis is a disability in itself. Additionally, it produces muscular imbalance that results in abnormal positions of joints, and also exposes the hand and foot to abnormal stresses which, in an anaesthetic limb, can cause destruction of deep tissues and ulceration of skin (Fig. 10.5). In disease in which paralysis occurs without anaesthesia, the patient still cares for his limbs and preserves them from injury. In leprosy, paralysis serves to accentuate and aggravate the effects of anaesthesia. A common example is seen in a claw hand (Fig. 10.6). When the patient grasps a tool the interphalangeal joints are hyper-flexed, and excessive pressure is exerted at the tips of the fingers. The subcuticular pulp is bruised against the sharp tips of the phalanges. Repeated bruising destroys the pulp. The skin becomes callous, impinges directly on bone and soon ulcerates.

A hand that functions poorly is not fully used; tendons shorten and joints become stiff. Stiff joints are, however, more commonly due to damage from misuse, ulceration, secondary infection and fibrous ankylosis.

With paralysis of intrinsic muscles of the foot, the toes become hyperextended at the metatarsophalangeal joints and are clawed. There is less muscular protection over the metatarsal heads, which become prone to injury, and the skin over them to ulceration. Drop

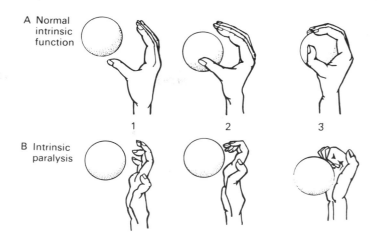

Fig. 10.5 Stages of grasp in normal and claw hands.

A1. A normal hand opens with extension of all finger joints.

A2. Closure is begun by pure intrinsic muscle action with flexion of metacarpophalangeal joints; interphalangeal joints remain extended.

A3. Grasping the object is completed by long flexor action at the interphalangeal joints.

B1. With intrinsic muscle paralysis, hyperextension of metacarpophalangeal joints may partially compensate for flexion of interphalangeal joints.

B2. Closure is begun and completed by the long flexors which roll the fingers shut from their tips.

B3. A large object cannot be grasped. A small object is grasped between the finger tips and the metacarpal heads.

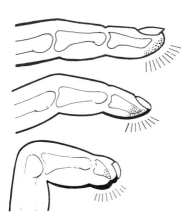

Fig. 10.6 Mechanism of damage in anaesthetic paralysed finger. Repetitive trauma to a clawed and anaesthetic finger tip causes callus and subcuticular destruction of pulp and of the tip of the distal phalanx.

foot makes walking difficult, and if there is anaesthesia the forefoot ulcerates readily.

4. Misuse

At least nine out of ten injuries in anaesthetic hands and feet follow from misuse. Misuse of an anaesthetic limb allows injury to take place without the patient realizing it. The injury is neglected, complications set in, and the vicious cycle of tissue destruction and disability has begun. In this way minor injuries become major disasters. The nature of the injury will depend to some extent upon the age, sex, occupation and customs of the patient: an office worker wearing stylish shoes, which may well be too tight, will be more prone to friction blisters and less to cuts and puncture wounds than will a barefoot farmer. A housewife is especially liable to burn her hands while cooking.

Six types of injury are common. Those due to repeated, prolonged or excessive force are most important.

a. Bruises from minimal repeated trauma. Bruising follows the excessive repetition or over-vigorous performance of a normal function, such as walking or handling a tool. The pressure needed to produce the bruise is in the range 1.4–3.5 kg/cm^2. But it must be repeated many thousands of times. The first few thousand repetitions produce inflammation, which is painful in a normal limb and limits activity. In an anaesthetic limb there is no such limitation. The next few thousand repetitions cause necrosis of the inflamed part and haemorrhage into it. If the bruise is recognized, even at this stage, and the part is rested, ulceration can be prevented and healing may take place without scar formation. Further episodes of bruising can be prevented if the activity causing them is restricted and if new types of repetitive activities are introduced gradually, thereby allowing time for tissues to hypertrophy and so to withstand stresses that would not normally be tolerated.

If the bruise is not recognized, subcutaneous tissue or even bone may be destroyed. Dead subcutaneous tissue and blood clot liquify and track of the side of the foot as a necrosis blister. The overlying skin may ulcerate (Fig. 10.7). Such an ulcer used to be called, incorrectly, a trophic ulcer. The bones most likely to sustain damage by this process are the metatarsals. There is aseptic necrosis and absorption of the heads and concentric absorption of the shafts, which become narrowed and pointed like a pencil, with thickening of cortical bone (Fig. 10.8).

In the foot there are two types of force which, when repeatedly applied, cause bruising and ulceration. They are termed 'thrust' and

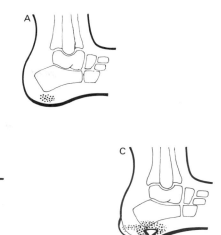

Fig. 10.7   Stages in the development of plantar ulceration in an anaesthetic foot.
A. Repetitive stress bruises subcutaneous tissues.
B. If it is not allowed to heal, bruising leads to necrosis. The liquified debris tracks to the surface as a necrosis blister, either directly under the bruise or sideways to the softer glabrous skin at the edge of the sole, as shown here. The blister remains sterile so long as the skin is not broken.
C. The skin breaks down, producing an ulcer which may be at the site of the blister or directly overlying the bony prominence, as shown here. Sometimes the ulcer extends to include both sites.

'shear'. 'Thrust' is a direct blunt force, whose effects have been described above. 'Shear' is the force pulling at the subcutaneous tissues as the foot is in motion during walking or running. As the foot touches the ground, the skin is pulled back; as the foot pushes off from the ground the skin is pulled forward. This motion is not dangerous in a normal foot, as pain warns if too much force is exerted. In the scarred foot the subcutaneous tissues cannot slide normally and shear may be excessive; if the foot is anaesthetic, more subcutaneous tissue is broken down and ulceration follows.

b. Necrosis from prolonged or abnormal pressures. Mild pressure, as little as 0.07 kg/cm^2, can cause necrosis and ulceration if constantly applied for several hours. Such pressure may be exerted by a tight shoe or by a bandage within a shoe as is commonly worn by a patient with an ulcer on the foot. Patients with deformed feet sometimes wear ready-made, but ill-fitting shoes in order to hide their deformity. Other examples of situations where prolonged and constant, but slight pressure can cause tissue necrosis are gripping a hand rail while travelling on a bus or leaning

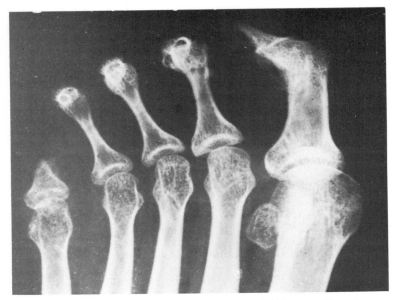

Fig. 10.8 Radiograph of forefoot, borderline tuberculoid leprosy. There is osteoporosis of metatarsal heads and loss of medullary markings and cortical definition. There is some tapering of metatarsal shafts and cortical sclerosis of their necks. The shafts of the proximal phalanges are markedly narrowed. This damage is due to repeated excessive trauma while walking on an anaesthetic foot. The toes are clawed, because of intrinsic muscle paralysis, which has allowed trauma to damage or destroy the distal phalanges. Lateral deviation of the toes is a result of muscular imbalance.

on an elbow while playing a game of chess. In these examples, lack of pain in an anaesthetic limb deprives the patient of the warning to change his stance, grip or posture.

The adverse effects of constant pressure are accentuated by pre-existing deformity, which may allow pressure to bear upon sites which are not protected by a fibro-fatty subcutaneous pad. In this situation pressures may be greatly increased. For example, a pair of normal hands, lifting a 22.5 kg block, experiences a pressure of 0.2 kg/cm². The same weight, taken on the tip of clawed fingers exerts a pressure of 2.1 kg/cm², which rapidly kills tissue.

A patient with an anaesthetic hand does not know how much force is required to hold an object, such as a tool or key, in order to execute a particular action, and, therefore, does so with maximum force, exerting much more pressure than is necessary. A blunt object will bruise and a sharp one may cut the skin.

c. Puncture wounds and cuts. Penetration of the skin by thorns, nails or other sharp pointed objects frequently produces a wound that does not bleed, nor produce obvious skin damage, and is not readily noticed in an anaesthetic limb. A normal person will stop walking and remove a thorn from his foot because it hurts, but a person who feels no pain will continue to walk. The wound fills with dirt and every step drives infection deeper into the tissues. Fever, painful inguinal lymphadenitis or gross swelling of the foot make the patient realize his precarious situation. Otherwise necrosis and ulceration are inevitable.

Cuts are more easily recognized than puncture wounds because they bleed or may be seen; but, if neglected because of anaesthesia, cuts lead to equally serious complications.

d. Burns. Burns are a common form of injury. An anaesthetic hand fails to recognize, or recognizes too late, the heat of a cooking pot or cigarette; an anaesthetic foot painlessly treads on a red-hot ember or steps into a too-hot bath (Fig. 10.9). Many leprosy patients, and even some doctors, think that leprosy itself commonly causes blisters on the hands and feet. Such blisters are almost always due to burns, or to friction. Very occasionally erythema nodosum leprosum may produce blisters around the margin of the sole or palm.

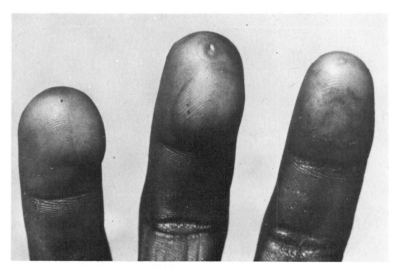

Fig. 10.9 Trauma in an anaesthetic hand. The blisters on the middle and ring fingers followed a burn caused by lifting a hot cooking pot. The scarring at the tips of the index and middle fingers resulted from repetitive minor trauma to clawed anaesthetic fingers (Fig. 10.6).

Second degree burns heal without scarring if they are properly treated and infection is excluded; but third degree burns may cause extensive loss of tissue and scar formation.

 e. Blisters due to friction. The wearing of a shoe that is too loose or the repetitive use of a tool held in the hand may cause a blister. Normally the blister is painful; the patient stops his activity and the blister heals. Anaesthesia delays recognition of the blister and further activity leads to ulceration.

 f. Dislocation of joints. An uncommon, but severely disabling, injury may follow from loss of two types of sensation in and around a joint: stretch and pain. If a normal person twists his ankle while walking, tendons are stretched and reflex muscle contraction splints the joint. At the same time reflex relaxation of muscles around the knee and hip takes the weight off that ankle. The person stumbles, but the joint is saved. Loss of sensation to stretch and pain allows the person to put his full weight on the turned ankle, ligaments are torn and the joint becomes unstable. Further walking causes dislocation and even fractures, thus producing the disorganized or neuropathic joint. The

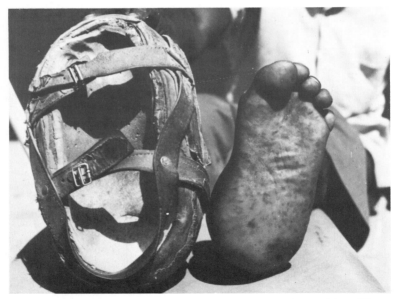

Fig. 10.10 A simple orthopaedic shoe can protect a badly damaged foot. The foot has lost its arches and the toes are clawed and deviated. In the past there have been many plantar ulcers. The skin is kept healthy now because the shoe, which is made of microcellular rubber built up beneath a moulded Plastazote® insole, distributes the weight evenly all over the sole of the foot (Fig. 12.4).

first clinical evidence of injury is swelling and heat around the ankle. By comparison with the other foot it may be seen that the medial arch is flattened (Fig. 10.10). A radiograph of the bones will define the problem. Commonly the injury results in a collapse of the neck of the talus (Fig. 10.11).

5. Ulceration

Any of the six types of injury sustained as a result of misuse of anaesthetic limbs may cause or lead to ulceration. Of the six, bruising from repeated minimal traumas is the most important. Plantar ulceration is possibly the commonest secondary complication in leprosy. The commonest sites of plantar ulceration are over the metatarsal heads, the base of the fifth metatarsal, the base of the proximal phalanx and the calcaneus. Ulceration is damaging because it permits secondary infection and heals by scar formation (Fig. 10.12).

6. Scar formation

Defects caused by ulceration are replaced by scar tissue which is weaker and has a poorer supply than has healthy tissue. As the scar

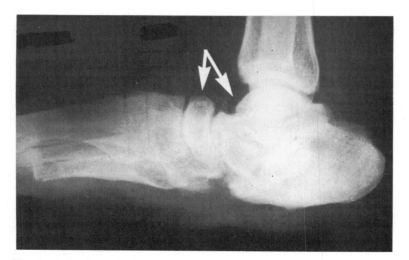

Fig. 10.11 Radiograph of foot shown in Figure 10.11, showing tarsal damage. In this patient, repeated trauma has caused increased density and partial collapse of the talus and navicular bones (arrowed), with the development of dorsal lips. The calcaneum is also flattened. A well-designed shoe will distribute weight evenly and prevent further damage from walking.

contracts, the blood supply becomes still poorer and the scar may break down as a result of minor injury, or even spontaneously. Scars distort the hand or foot, cause an abnormal distribution of pressure, and encourage further ulceration.

7. Secondary infection

Just as anaesthesia delays recognition of mechanical injury so also it delays recognition of infection that so commonly complicates injury. Cellulitis develops and destroys subcutaneous tissue, and infection may reach bone. The patient is fortunate if systemic symptoms arise forcing him to recognize that something is wrong; but by that time permanent damage may be inevitable.

Osteomyelitis causes much greater damage to bone than does aseptic necrosis following repeated traumata, osteoporosis following disuse or erosion following direct invasion by *M. leprae*. In many patients these mechanisms co-exist. As a result of osteomyelitis, bone is absorbed, sequestra are extruded, and the architecture of the foot or hand is irretrievably distorted (Figs 10.12, 10.13). But even these late changes can be halted by controlling infection, preventing further trauma, and allowing overlying tissues to heal.

The sequence of events, from anaesthesia to disability, is also found in other conditions which cause loss of sensation, such as diabetes, tabes dorsalis, syringomyelia and spina bifida. In leprosy there may be additional disability resulting from invasion of tissues by *M. leprae*.

8. Invasion of tissues by M. leprae

In lepromatous leprosy all the tissues of the hands and feet may be infiltrated with *M. leprae*, and may not function normally. Bones may fracture (see p. 36 and Fig. 4.13). Reactional inflammation may increase tissue damage and be followed by stiff joints, and so contribute to the disability.

Prevention of disability

The sequence of events which leads from nerve damage to disability can be interrupted at four points (Fig. 10.14):

1. Prevention of misuse, by protecting anaesthetic limbs and by teaching the patient how to care for them.

2. Early recognition of inflammation, so that the part may be rested before ulceration takes place.

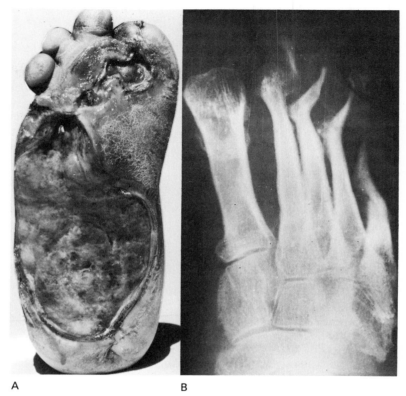

A   B

Fig. 10.12 a Loss of tissue in an anaesthetic foot. The sole of the foot is
anaesthetic (posterior tibial nerve damage). The unusual size and position of the
ulcer is due to loss of architecture following extensive *previous damage* the foot
has sustained. The skin over the heel is pulled in by scar tissue binding it down
to the calcaneus causing loss of skin movement and increasing susceptibility to
shear forces. *Abnormal pressures* over the 3rd, 4th and 5th metatarsal heads have
destroyed them and damage to the posterior tibial nerve has led to intrinsic
paralysis, clawing, increased pressure, ulceration of toes, osteomyelitis and
destruction of phalanges.

b Radiograph of the foot shown in **a**. Metatarsals are tapered due to repeated
trauma and infection, and their heads are lost. The metatarsophalangeal
joints are dislocated and useless. The phalanges are mere ghosts.
Such severe loss of architecture renders the anaesthetic foot liable to repeated
ulceration. The damage here results from *anaesthesia*, *misuse* and *secondary
osteomyelitis*.

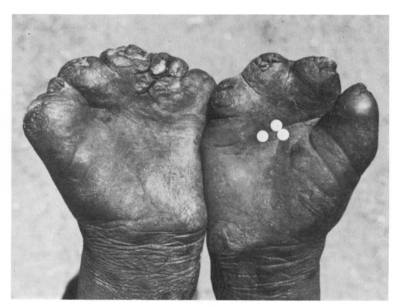

Fig. 10.13 Too late! This tragic sight is all too common at leprosy clinics. Dapsone cannot restore lost fingers.

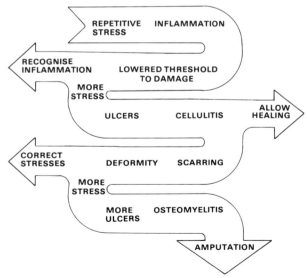

Fig. 10.14 The downhill path which leads from nerve damage to deformity and amputation. The path may be avoided by preventing misuse, and may be left at three places (adapted from the original by Dr Paul Brand).

3. Permitting ulceration to heal as soon as it is detected, so that there is a minimum of residual scarring and distortion.

4. Providing protection for damaged hands and feet, in order to distribute pressure evenly and to prevent further injury.

FURTHER READING

Brand P W 1981 Insensitive feet, a practical handbook on foot problems in leprosy. The Leprosy Mission, London

Brand P W Repetitive stress on insensitive feet, Pamphlet — US Pub Health Service, Carville, La., 70721, U.S.A.

Coleman W C, Madrigal D R 1985 The patient with sensory loss. International Journal of Leprosy 53: 255–257

Fritschi E P 1987 Field detection of early neuritis in leprosy. Leprosy Review 58: 173–177

Karat S, Karat A B A, Foster R 1968 Radiological changes in bones of the limbs in leprosy. Leprosy Review 39: 147–169

Naafs B, Dagne T 1977 Sensory testing: a sensitive method in the follow up of nerve involvement. International Journal of Leprosy 45: 364–368

Paterson D E, Job C K 1964 Bone changes and absorption in leprosy. In: Cochrane R G, Davey R F (eds) Leprosy in theory and practice. Wright, Bristol, pp. 425–446

Watson J M 1986 Preventing disability in leprosy patients. The Leprosy Mission International, London

11. The eye in leprosy

Blindness is a common and disastrous complication of leprosy. Coming on top of anaesthesia of hands and feet it is nothing less than a calamity, further limiting communication of the patient with the world about him. Eye-damage in leprosy often starts insidiously and the patient may not mention that his sight is not quite as good as it used to be or that he commonly has a little pain in one eye. Examination of the eye is an important part of the examination of any patient who is suspected of having leprosy and a re-examination should be routine at each revisit. Ten minutes well spent can prevent years of blindness. The differential diagnosis of eye lesions is considered on page 75.

EXAMINATION OF THE EYE*

Look at the face to see if there is any evidence of a lesion near or around the eye. Lepromatous infiltration of the face or a large tuberculoid patch encircling the eye indicate danger of conjunctival infiltration, anaesthesia or paralysis. Look at the lids for ectropion or entropion and see that they move fully when the patient blinks.

Ask the patient to close his eyes, gently at first and then firmly, and see if he can keep them closed for 10 seconds. This will show lagophthalmos which threatens damage from exposure. Feel the intraocular tension with the tips of both index fingers or if possible use a tonometer.

Look at the conjunctivae for lepromatous infiltration and for perilimbal injection which is a sign of iridocyclitis. See if the surface of the cornea is moist and that the tears are draining properly through the puncta. See if the pupil will contract normally and regularly to light.

Look carefully at the surface of the cornea and of the iris, and at the margin of the pupil. This is best done with a corneal microscope, but if

---

*For definitions of ophthalmological terms see p. 162 and Figure 11.1.

153

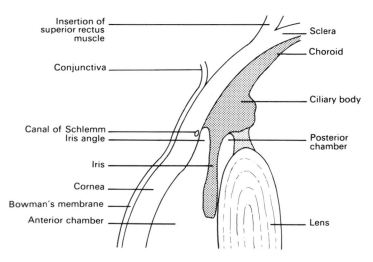

Fig. 11.1   Longitudinal section of the upper anterior quadrant of the eye.

that is not available a substitute can be made using the beam of a well focused torch, which is shone on to the eye obliquely, and a corneal loupe (hand lens with magnification x 8 or greater). These two features are incorporated in Hobbs illuminated slit loupe. Examine the fundus with an ophthalmoscope for the presence of lesions due to other diseases.

Finally, measure visual acuity with a Snellen test chart. If the patient is illiterate the multiple *E* chart is used. If vision is impaired, find out why.

WAYS IN WHICH THE EYE CAN BE DAMAGED

Exposure and anaesthesia

Damage to the seventh nerve is common in leprosy and it is particularly the occipito-temporal and zygomatic branches which are affected, producing a selective paralysis of the orbicularis oculi muscle (Fig. 4.20). The most superficial fibres of the muscle are often most severely paralysed. This can happen in any type of leprosy but is especially common in association with tuberculoid (TT or BT) lesions of the face, especially during type 1 reactions, and in late untreated lepromatous leprosy. Bacillary infiltration of the superficial muscles of the face may contribute to the weakness in lepromatous leprosy. Lagophthalmos results, blinking is incomplete and the cornea and conjunctiva become prone to drying and to minor traumata. Reactions of tuberculoid lesions of the face may result in scarring of the tarsal plate with the development of entropion and trichiasis. Both these events are disastrous if there is anaesthesia.

Damage to the ophthalmic branch of the fifth nerve results in anaesthesia of the cornea and conjunctiva. This can happen when a tuberculoid patch covers the eye or when there is lepromatous invasion of corneal nerves. Partial loss of corneal sensation and drying of the cornea are often interpreted as 'itch'. The patient may easily injure such an eye by rubbing it. With more profound anaesthesia the incentive to blink is lost and exposure and trauma rapidly cause ulceration of the cornea which, if not vigorously treated, perforates and the eye becomes blind.

Bacillary invasion

In lepromatous leprosy the eye is invaded through the bloodstream.

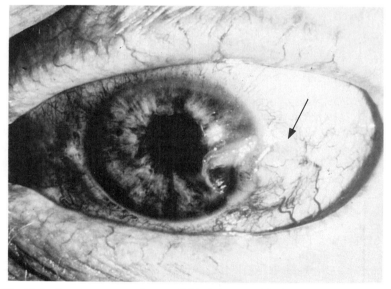

Fig. 11.2   Eye, lepromatous leprosy (LL). A large nodule is seen lateral to the limbus with vessels coursing around and over it (arrowed). The eye is in reaction and there is circumlimbal injection. There is an ulcer on the cornea adjacent to the nodule. Ulceration often occurs where a swelling overrides the cornea and prevents normal tear distribution by the lids. The iris margin is irregular and frayed, indicating many previous attacks of iridocyclitis. In attempting surgical removal of the nodule it was found that it continued deep into the sclera and probably originated in the ciliary body.

Lepromatoa may form on the conjunctiva and infiltration extends onto the cornea (Fig. 11.2). Bacilli multiply in the ciliary body which is rendered extremely susceptbile to reactions. The effects of bacillary invasion and hypersenstitivity are far more severe in Mongolians and Caucasians than in Negroes.

Hypersensitivity

Tissues of the eye that have been invaded by leprosy bacilli are liable to severe damage during type 2 reactions. This is especially true of the iris and ciliary body. It is also possible that they may be the site of deposition of circulating immune complexes even when there are no bacilli there. The inflammation of iridocyclitis causes synechiae, fixing the iris to the lens (posterior) or cornea (anterior). Posterior synechiae or plugging of the pupil with inflammatory exudate may obstruct the flow of aqueous from the posterior chamber. Extensive anterior synechiae may, on occasion, prevent the flow of aqueous into the Canal of Schlemm. Either of these processes causes glaucoma, which may be followed by optic atrophy and blindness.

CLINICAL FEATURES

Exposure and anaesthesia

If *lagophthalmos* is not treated, the superficial fibres of the orbicularis oculi muscle fibrose and shorten, and the deep fibres exert uneven pressure on the tarsal plate everting the lid and causing *ectropion* which increases exposure. Both cornea and conjunctiva undergo chronic changes as a result of the drying due to exposure. The puncta no longer touch the conjunctiva, and tears flow over the face.

Anaesthesia is sought by lightly touching the cornea with a wisp of cotton wool with the patient looking upwards and away from the examining hand. Normal sensation is indicated by immediate and brisk blink reflex. *Corneal ulceration* may at first be superficial and only detectable with a loupe. If the cornea is anaesthetic the ulcer is not painful and is only recognized because of lacrimation and conjunctival inflammation. The ulcer may heal leaving a scar which interferes with vision or else it becomes infected and penetrates to the back of the cornea (Fig. 11.2). An active ulcer can be distinguished from a healed scar after instillation of 1% fluorescein. Inflammatory debris collects in the anterior chamber with the formation of *hypopyon*. If the process is not arrested infection penetrates the eye which then becomes blind.

Infection of the lacrimal sac is a constant source of danger to the eye. When there is lagophthalmos, apply pressure over the lacrimal sac and see if the puncta exude pus — a sign of dacryocystitis.

Bacillary invasion

The first signs are beading of corneal nerves which can be seen only with the corneal microscope. Lepromatous infiltration of the corneal surface starts as a punctate keratitis with discrete small white opacities, usually of the upper temporal quadrant, which may fuse resulting in a general haze of Bowman's membrane. This punctate keratitis is pathognomonic of leprosy (Fig. 11.3). Some of these opacities calcify, become more dense and are called corneal pearls. Punctate keratitis may cross the centre of the cornea and cause hazy vision. Later, pannus is laid down; this seldom reaches the centre of the cornea and usually causes no symptoms.

Early lepromatous bacillary invasion of the conjunctiva cannot be seen, but smears will contain acid-fast bacilli. Later a lepromatous

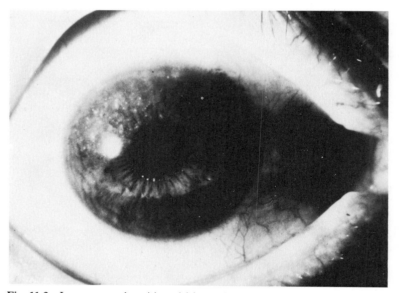

Fig. 11.3   Lepromatous keratitis and iris pearls. This is the right eye of a patient with lepromatous leprosy. It shows superficial punctate keratitis with scarring of Bowman's membrane which looks like a light haze covering the upper temporal quadrant of the cornea. The chalky white spots seen against this haze are lepromata which have become degenerate and calcified — corneal pearls. Similar pearls are seen on the iris at the lower pupillary margin.

nodule may appear on the conjunctiva as a small yellow mass, usually on the exposed part of the limbus, and can interfere with lid closure or become the site of a reaction (Fig. 11.2). It must be distinguished from a pterygium.

Iris pearls, comparable to those in the cornea, may be the only visible sign of invasion of the uveal tract, but by the time they appear the whole of the anterior segment of the eye is invaded including the choroid, ciliary body and sclera. There may be no symptoms until a reaction starts.

Hypersensitivity and its complications

Iridocyclitis

The most important manifestation of type 2 reactions in the eye is acute iridocyclitis (Figs 11.2, 11.4). It is the most frequent cause of blindness in leprosy. It causes:

Pain, which is felt deep in the eye and is severe enough to make the patient seek help. Patients who have lost ocular sensation are often unaware of pain as a warning symptom. The other symptoms should,

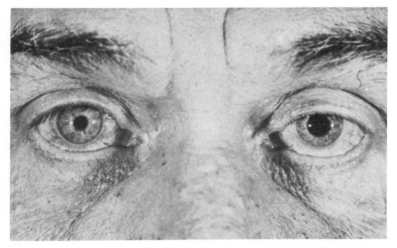

Fig. 11.4 Iridocyclitis. The right eye shows perilimbal injection and a smaller pupil than its fellow. This picture was taken early in an attack of iridocyclitis in a patient with active lepromatous leprosy complicated by intermittent iridocyclitis. Atropine drops were used to dilate the pupils because the condition was bilateral. The left pupil responds better than the right, which is also slightly irregular due to posterior synechiae.

therefore, be explained to the patient so that he will be alert to early inflammation.

Photophobia with increased lacrimation.

Blurring of vision and diminution in visual acuity.

'*Pink eye*' in which the inflammation is around the limbus rather than over the whole of the conjunctiva as in conjunctivitis.

Constriction of the pupil which does not respond readily to light and which may be irregular. If there have been previous attacks the iris may be thin and have lost its regular pattern; its edge is frayed and the pupil distorted, and fragments of iris may be seen stuck to the lens.

Cloudiness of the anterior chamber is due to inflammatory exudation of white cells floating in the aqueous humour. This is the very earliest sign of iridocyclitis. It often causes the patient little or no discomfort, and unfortunately is only detected with the use of the slit-lamp microscope. These cells form keratic precipitates on the back of the cornea.

After several attacks of acute iridocyclitis a state of subacute or chronic inflammation may persist, and symptoms may be minimal. Careful examination of the eye including a test of visual acuity is needed to detect the condition and prevent complications.

Iridocyclitis is typically only part of a generalized type 2 reaction and other manifestations such as erythema nodosum leprosum and painful neuritis (see Ch. 8) are usually present too. Occasionally however an attack of iridocyclitis may be the first sign of lepromatous leprosy.

Scleritis and episcleritis

Sometimes the coats of the eyeball rather than the uveal tract are the site of a reaction which produces a patch of tender hyperaemia visible through the conjunctiva. Chronic inflammation may weaken the sclera so that the pigmented choroid herniates through as a staphyloma.

Synechiae

Attachment of the iris to the surface of the lens or cornea deforms and tears the pupil and this is clearly seen when the pupil is dilated with a mydriatic. Other signs of chronic iris damage are often present. One of the main purposes in treating iridocyclitis is to prevent synechiae.

Glaucoma

This is a common complication of recurrent iridocyclitis. The conjunctiva becomes dusky pink and the tension of the eyeball is raised. Visual acuity is reduced and in late cases there is pallor of the optic disc. Synechiae may be present, indicating past attacks of iridocyclitis. Pink eye in leprosy is commonly due to iridocyclitis, not glaucoma. If in doubt one should treat the iridocyclitis first. Many patients do not have symptoms until the intra-ocular pressure is high and vision is already impaired. Intraocular pressure should, therefore, be measured regularly in all patients with evidence of previous or current inflammation.

Cataract

This is another complication of recurrent iridocyclitis.

MANAGEMENT

Prevention

With early diagnosis and treatment the complications of eye disease should be preventable. Anaesthesia and damage from exposure need never occur and early lepromatous invasion can be halted. Even so, reactions may develop during treatment and the patient must be taught to attend regularly and to report at once any pain, blurring of vision or increased lacrimation.

Treatment

Treatment of exposure and anaesthesia

Massage and exercise. Massage and active forced closure of the lids and facial muscles may restore enough tone after a few months to permit lid closure in mild cases of lagophthalmos.

Prevent drying. Use a tear substitute. The best is a 1.4% solution of polyvinyl alcohol (PVA) in water. This is expensive but hospitals with a prosthetics department may have scraps of PVA sheeting. These are dissolved in sterile water with gentle heat and 1% chlorbutanol is added as a preservative. One drop should be instilled thrice daily. Alternatively during the day 1% methylcellulose or 1% sodium bicarbonate drops are suitable substitutes for tears. At night sterile castor oil or petrolatum can be used.

Protect against injury. Spectacles with plain or tinted lenses should be worn by day. Goggles may be needed at work if there is danger from flying particles of metal or wood.

Control secondary infection. Daily instillation of 1% zinc sulphate in 4% boric acid helps. Infection of the lacrimal sac requires more vigorous treatment with local and systemic antibiotics.

Patients with lagophthalmos which cannot be corrected by conservative measures, or which is complicated by corneal anaesthesia or pre-existing corneal damage, will require surgery. The common procedures used, tarsorrhaphy and temporalis tendon transfer are described on page 176.

Treatment of bacillary invasion

Whenever there is direct invasion of the eye with leprosy bacilli, antileprosy drugs should be given in the usual way (see p. 85). Bacilli may persist in the eye for many years after they have been eliminated from the skin.

Conjunctival lepromata should be shaved down with a scalpel if they prevent approximation of the lid to the cornea during blinking.

Treatment of hypersensitivity (type 2) reactions:

Reaction in the eye will usually be part of a general type 2 reaction which may demand systemic anti-inflammatory treatment (see p. 128). Certain local measures are required specifically for ocular involvement.

1. Acute iridocyclitis. Dilate the pupil and relax the ciliary muscle by instilling atropine 1% or scopolamine 0.25% as drops or ointment. This is done thrice daily at first and then daily for as long as inflammation persists. A stronger mydriatic which is used to free synechiae in severe or recurrent cases is mydricaine (atropine sulphate 0.016 g, cocaine 0.03 g, adrenaline 1: 1000 3 ml, distilled water 6 ml; the adrenaline is added after sterilization). This is given by subconjunctival injection into the fornix, in a dose of 0.2 ml daily for four days, after anaesthetizing the cornea with cocaine. Thereafter the acute process can usually be controlled by daily use of atropine ointment or drops. Atropine, by paralysing the iris, causes photophobia and the patient may benefit from the use of dark glasses.

Suppress inflammation by the instillation of 1% cortisone or hydrocortisone every 4 hours. Alternatively, or in severe cases additionally, a subconjunctival injection is given of 0.2 ml of a solution containing 25 mg of hydrocortisone per ml (preparations made up for intra-articular injection are suitable) or of 10 mg of methylprednisolone.

Relieve pain. Pain will stop as the inflammation subsides, but can be helped by giving aspirin 600 mg four hourly and by steaming the eye over a cloth-covered spoon which is repeatedly dipped in boiling water.

Reconsider the chemotherapy. If iridocyclitis persists consider a change to clofazimine (see p. 130)

2. Chronic iridocyclitis and scleritis. Treatment with local instillation of atropine and hydrocortisone is maintained for months or years, each being given once daily. It is necessary to check tension for rising intra-ocular pressure at regular intervals and to tell the patient to report any increase of pain as this could indicate the onset of glaucoma. Treatment is continued until no cells can be seen in the anterior chamber through the slit lamp, or for three months longer than it takes for all symptoms and signs of inflammation to subside.

3. Treatment of complications of reactions.

Glaucoma. In leprosy glaucoma is a complication of iridocyclitis, and one for which treatment must be maintained. Additionally, acetazolamide 250 mg is given orally thrice daily. Iridectomy may be indicated if the response is poor.

Cataract. Cataracts may be removed from a quiet eye, but in the knowledge that a reaction may be precipitated, for which reason it is wise to give a pre-operative subconjunctival injection of 20 mg methyl prednisolone. Eyes which are or have in the previous six months been inflamed should not be operated upon.

OPHTHALMOLOGICAL DEFINITIONS

Anterior chamber. Portion of aqueous space in front of the iris.

Anterior segment. Anterior third of eye, including the lens and ciliary body.

Bowman's membrane. The anterior, or superficial layer of the corneal stroma, just beneath the epithelium.

Cataract. Opacity of the lens.

Chemosis. Oedema of the conjunctiva.

Ciliary body. Root of the iris, containing muscles and blood vessels.

Dacryocystitis. Inflammation of the lacrimal sac.

Ectropion. Eversion of the edge of the eyelids.

Entropion. Inversion of the edge of eyelids.

Episcleritis. Inflammation of connective tissue overlying the sclera.

Glaucoma. Raised intra-ocular pressure and the syndrome arising from it.

Hypopyon. Accumulation of pus in the anterior chamber of eye.

Iridocyclitis. Inflammation of the iris and ciliary body: uveitis.

Keratic precipitates. Leucocytes, and other debris stuck on the posterior surface of the cornea.

Lagophthalmos. Incomplete closure of the eyelids.

Limbus. Junction of cornea with sclera and conjunctiva.

Madarosis. Loss of eyebrows or eyelashes, or both.

Mydriatic. Drug which dilates the pupil.

Pannus. Vascularization of the cornea.

Posterior chamber. Portion of the aqueous space behind the iris.

Pterygium. A triangular thickening of the perilimbal conjunctiva attached to the cornea and usually lateral to it.

Staphyloma. Protrusion or herniation of cornea or sclera.

Synechia. Attachment of the iris to lens (posterior) or cornea (anterior).

Tarsorrhaphy. Operation of suturing together a portion of the eyelids in order to reduce the width of the palpebral fissure.

Trichiasis. Ingrowing of the eyelashes.

FURTHER READING

Brand M E 1987 Care of the eye in Hansen's Disease. The Star, Carville, USA

Hobbs H E, Choyce D P 1971 The blinding lesions of leprosy. Leprosy Review 42: 131–137

Hobbs H E 1972 Leprotic iritis and blindness. International Journal of Leprosy 40: 366–374

Joffrion V C, Brand M E 1984 Leprosy of the eye — a general outline, Leprosy Review 55: 105–114

12. Physical rehabilitation

This chapter considers the practical procedures that may be needed to get a patient over the physical disabilities of leprosy, especially those resulting from nerve damage. In the most severely disabled the problems are great, but incentive and opportunity are often more important than physical capability. Even a person who is severely deformed and blind can still do useful work. It is psychologically important that after rehabilitation, each patient be as independent as possible.

PREVENTION OF PHYSICAL DISABILITY

It must be stressed again that the most important aspect of the management of leprosy is the prevention of anaesthesia and paralysis. This is achieved by:

1. Early diagnosis, before the nerves are irreparably damaged.
2. Early treatment to forestall nerve damage.
3. Judicious treatment, with great vigilance of patients with borderline leprosy.
4. Prompt recognition and vigorous treatment of reactions involving nerves and eyes.

In addition:

5. Convince the patient he need not be disabled, and teach him the danger signals of neuritis and iridocyclitis.

MANAGEMENT OF PHYSICAL DISABILITY

Control of ulceration

Plantar ulceration is the commonest serious disability in leprosy, and is of tremendous economic importance. It is essential to understand the genesis of ulceration in leprosy and to remember that the commonest cause of an ulcer is the *previous ulcer*.

Prevention of ulceration

Ulceration and destruction of extremities *can* be avoided. Patients can be educated in the care of anaesthetic parts, but first they must recognize and acknowledge their lack of normal sensation. Far too often patients are unwilling to admit to being abnormal.

Practices that should be implemented to help a person preserve his anaesthetic limbs are:

You yourself, as doctor or medical worker, show concern for the patient. Express interest in the patient's effort to preserve his limbs in spite of his inability to feel pain. It is important to him that he remain free of ulcers, but show that it is important to you as well.

Teach the patient to respect his hands and feet, to accept them as part of his body. Teach him to inspect daily for any trauma and to care for the smallest injury (Fig. 12.1).

Treat the first ulcer as the calamity that it is, and while treating, show that further ulcers need not occur. Show him how the injury is

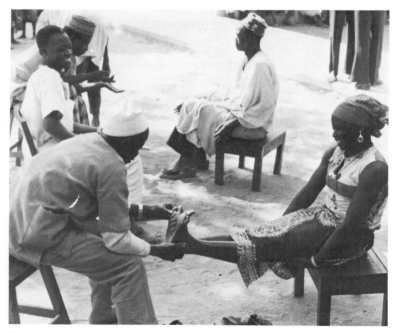

Fig. 12.1 Foot and hand clinic. Weekly inspection of anaesthetic feet and hands detects early damage and ensures that shoes are kept in good condition. Patients are taught to inspect their own hands, feet and shoes daily.

best treated, by using a mechanical splint to replace the splinting previously done by pain.

Help the patient to determine the cause of every injury. Never allow him to believe the damage is a result of 'leprosy'. Was it due to friction, a blow, a puncture, a burn? How and when did it occur? Only when he has understood the cause can he avoid future injury.

Protect anaesthetic feet with shoes. Without shoes there is no hope of staying free of ulcers. There are three principles in the design of shoes for anaesthetic feet:

1. Inner sole softness and elasticity, to protect compromised tissues.
2. Moulding the inner sole to the foot, to distribute weight evenly.
3. Firmness of the outer sole to provide protection and, for deformed feet, rigidity to prevent shearing.

The degree to which a shoe needs to be 'tailored' to the needs of the foot depends upon the extent of the abnormality. Feet can be considered in four categories depending upon the severity of the disability.

a. The low risk foot. The foot that is anaesthetic, with no or very minimal scarring.

b. The moderate risk foot. One that has multiple scars and some loss of the subcutaneous fat pad.

c. The high risk foot. One that has a mild deformity of the architecture such as flat foot, shortening or loss of digits.

d. The disintegrated foot. It has major bony deformity such as tarsal disintegration, the 'boat-shaped foot' or dislocation of the ankle.

a. *The low risk foot* needs protection and softness. A thin elastic sole inserted into a well-fitting shoe may be adequate for minor problems, but a thick insole may allow friction which can lead to ulceration. Sandals can be made with a sole of impervious material such as used car tyres and with an insole of microcellular rubber from 1 to 1.5 cm thick and of a softness that it can readily be compressed to half its thickness between thumb and finger. Straps can be cut from old inner tubes or split cords of tyres and their ends sewn between the two layers, through a slit in the outer sole (Fig. 12.2). Nails or wire must never be used.

b. *The moderate risk foot.* In addition to the above, the shoe should provide some moulding which can usually be done by adding a meta-tarsal bar and arch support so that the weight is partially taken from the area of the metatarsal heads, and distributed over the area of the arch. Alternatively, or in addition, moulding may be provided by making an insole of 1.25 cm formed polyethylene (e.g. Plastazote® —

I PROTECTION AND ELASTICITY

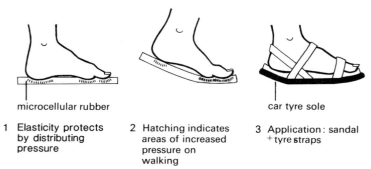

microcellular rubber   car tyre sole

1 Elasticity protects   2 Hatching indicates   3 Application: sandal
   by distributing   areas of increased   + tyre straps
   pressure   pressure on
                              walking

Fig. 12.2 Sandal for the low risk foot.

Smith & Nephew) which is moulded directly on to the foot. The patient stands on a sheet of Plastazote® that has been heated to exactly 140°C in an oven and is lying on a firm surface. Such footwear must have a heel counter and secure straps so that the foot remains in the proper position on the insole (Fig. 12.3).

   c. The high risk foot requires a sandal or preferably a shoe with more moulding and with a rigid sole. Moulding should conform completely to the abnormal contours of the foot. The patient stands on the heated Plastazote® which is lying on a layer of 10–150 cm foam rubber. The shoe is then built up under the Plastazote with layers of microcellular

II PROTECTION AND ELASTICITY AND MOULDING

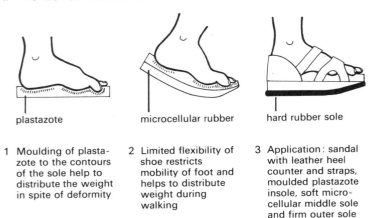

plastazote   microcellular rubber   hard rubber sole

1 Moulding of plasta-   2 Limited flexibility of   3 Application: sandal
   zote to the contours   shoe restricts   with leather heel
   of the sole help to   mobility of foot and   counter and straps,
   distribute the weight   helps to distribute   moulded plastazote
   in spite of deformity   weight during   insole, soft micro-
                             walking   cellular middle sole
                                                          and firm outer sole

Fig. 12.3 Sandal for the moderate risk foot.

III PROTECTION AND ELASTICITY AND MOULDING AND RIGIDITY

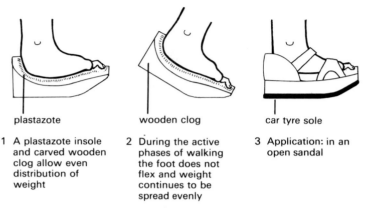

plastazote	wooden clog	car tyre sole
1 A plastazote insole and carved wooden clog allow even distribution of weight	2 During the active phases of walking the foot does not flex and weight continues to be spread evenly	3 Application: in an open sandal

Fig. 12.4 Sandal for the high risk foot.

rubber. A wooden rocker sole or hard rubber sole is fitted. Thus the moulded Plastazote® is applied to a wooden sole that has been carved to fit the undersurface of the Plastazote® accurately. The front of the wood block must be boat-shaped to provide 'rocker' action since the sole is rigid (Fig. 12.4). This shoe works well for the deformed and shortened foot.

d. The disintegrated foot is very difficult to rehabilitate. If there is a sub-talar destruction or dislocation of the ankle, it can occasionally be repaired by arthrodesis. If a stable plantigrade foot with reasonably good sole tissues can be obtained by surgery, the foot converts to type (c). If not, there is no alternative to amputation.

Nails or wire must *not* be used in shoes and sandals, which should be assembled with glue and sewn with nylon thread. The outward appearance of the shoe varies with the community. In some situations any shoe or sandal will be accepted. Elsewhere a particular style may indicate that its owner has leprosy, and so it must be made to look like a normal shoe, which makes the construction much more difficult.

A drop foot that is anaesthetic risks severe ulceration of the fore foot. A support should be added to the shoe (Fig. 12.5) or tendons transferred (p. 178).

A damaged and scarred foot that is adequately protected so that ulceration is prevented for a year or two will show a remarkable return towards normal. Scar tissue will soften and become supple. Depressed areas will fill in. Bone that was weakened by osteomyelitis and disuse

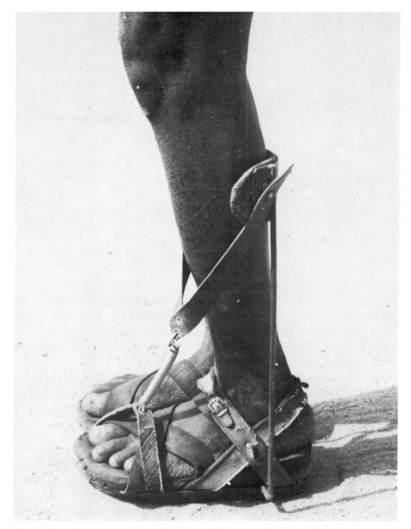

Fig. 12.5 Toe spring support for dropped foot. To a simple sandal (Fig. 12.2) are added two steel rods which are fixed to a padded steel plate at their upper ends, and which rotate in a metal bushing at their lower ends. A toe spring is attached by leather straps to complete the support.

atrophy will recalcify and callus will disappear completely. After this a simpler shoe may suffice.

Fissures of dry and anaesthetic feet and hands may be completely prevented by daily soaking for 30 minutes in water and then, after patting them dry, rubbing with petrolatum to prevent evaporation of water from the skin. Fissures that are already established are treated by paring away the thick callus with a blade or rubbing it down with a pumice stone to allow the skin to become soft so that the fissure may heal.

Hands that are dry, calloused or have deformities need to be protected during hard work. Some people suggest the adaptation of tool handles to prevent injury, but this is not acceptable to all patients; some refuse to use tools that are 'different'. An alternative that is acceptable in some communities is the use of a canvas work glove.

Restrict the use of anaesthetic parts. For many people the farming season brings added threat to both hands and feet. Walking to the farm and the extra trauma of farm work increase the risk of injury. Patients need to be helped to find ways of preventing injury. Gloves, or a cloth wrapped around tool handles, or restriction of the type or amount of actual work are possibilities. Some patients may need to seek another occupation, if that is possible. Where travel is a necessity some means of transport other than by foot is essential. A donkey may be cheaper than a bicycle and as satisfactory.

Management of ulceration

Ulceration is essentially due to mechanical factors and the management is essentially mechanical, by protecting the limb completely against these factors.

Of first importance is the care of minimal injury. Any skin break should be covered to prevent secondary infection and be splinted to allow healing to take place.

Ulceration can be healed by immobilization. After secondary infection has been controlled the foot is measured for a shoe and the limb is immobilized in a weight-bearing plaster cast for six weeks. Plaster casts applied on insensitive legs need special care. Padding should be applied only around the malleoli and across the front of the ankle. A felt strip down the front of the tibia makes removal easier. A thin layer of plaster is applied to the leg and moulded meticulously into every hollow until set. Then a back slab and reinforcing layers are added, and a Bohler iron or a plywood sole with rubber heel are attached. When the cast is taken off the shoe is ready for wear.

An alternative method of immobilization is by bed rest and crutches plus the application of a splint to prevent movement in an ulcer close to a joint. Not even *one* weight-bearing step is taken until complete healing has taken place and suitable footwear has been provided. When the patient starts to walk, he should walk only short distances and with small steps, to minimize the danger from shear forces or an inflamed scar.

If a patient is obliged to resume walking before the ulcer is completely healed, and his footwear has been made, the ulcer should be covered with a single layer of adhesive zinc oxide strapping. Ulcers will often continue to heal. Gauze dressings must never be worn in shoes as they increase pressure over the spot that should be protected.

Secondary infection should be controlled by systemic antibiotics, if it is deep or severe. Superficial infection is best treated with a topical antiseptic. Silver nitrate, 0.5% in water, is satisfactory as it prevents the growth of all, even antibiotic resistant, organisms. The solution can be made up with tap water if there are no minerals in the water that will precipitate the silver. Dressings must be changed twice daily and covered with a plastic film to prevent drying.

Debridement. Any dead tissues or callus should be removed. This is best done after the skin has been softened by soaking in water.

Skin grafting. Plantar ulcers, especially those that have recurred repeatedly or are extensively scarred, can be satisfactorily treated by complete excision of the ulcerated area and all scar tissue followed by splint skin grafting. This will provide a more suitable bed for regrowth of subcutaneous tissue than that provided by scar tissue. With protective shoes and due care on the part of the patient such a graft will give good coverage and will not break down again.

Recurrent ulceration in a foot that is being properly cared for suggests the presence of an underlying abnormality such as a bone spur, deep scarring, or lack of adequate subcutaneous tissue, especially over the metatarsal heads. Bone spurs can be removed, scar tissue excised, and tendons transferred to correct clawing of toes. A deep ulcer under the calcaneum heals with difficulty. The ulcer may be excised through a 'fish mouth' incision around the margin of the sole. The plantar defect is sutured in two layers before inserting a drain and suturing the 'fish mouth'.

Use of physiotherapy

Physiotherapy is an essential part of medical and surgical management in leprosy.

When nerves are invaded in leprosy, cellular exudate and oedema cause swelling within the relatively inflexible sheath, and this leads to ischaemia. Partial ischaemia causes neuropraxia, or impairment of conduction. If ischaemia is prolonged, the nerve is destroyed, but if blood flow can be restored promptly the nerve recovers and function returns.

Physiotherapy may be of help in preserving the physiological properties of paralysed muscles and preventing atrophy, as well as strengthening them during recovery. Even though nerve conduction may be impaired for a long time, some function may yet return. It is therefore imperative to maintain muscle bulk and activity during the period of paralysis. Physiotherapy should start as soon as possible in order to obtain a good result.

Paralysis is treated in two phases:

The expectant phase — when there is no sign of recovery having begun.

The active phase — when there is some return of nerve conduction.

The aims of physiotherapy in these phases are:

The expectant phase

    a. To prevent contracture and retain full range of movement.
    b. To prevent muscle atrophy.
    c. To prevent overstretching of paralysed muscles.

The means of attaining these aims are:

Assessment of nerve and muscle function. The methods are described in Chapter 10.

Passive movement. All joints that have been immobilized by paralysis are moved passively through the full range of motion each day.

Massage. Light massage of the affected muscles may help to maintain circulation and muscle tone.

Electrical stimulation. Faradic stimulation of paralysed muscles will help maintain tone and prevent atrophy, and should be done twice daily.

Splinting. All joints which cannot be maintained in the position of function by the patient should be splinted to prevent stretching of paralysed muscles and shortening of antagonists.

The active phase

The aim is to regain as much normal muscle power and range of movement as possible. The means of attaining this aim are:

1. Carefully graded exercises to strengthen the affected muscles.

2. Practising skilled co-ordinated movements such as those the patient will do on return to his former life and occupation.

A patient should do exercises as soon as the acute symptoms of neuritis have subsided. Exercises should be performed during three to five daily sessions, in each of which each exercise should be repeated 30 times. The patient begins with passive exercises; as function returns active exercises are introduced.

Hands. For lumbrical paralysis, the seated patient places his affected hand palm upward on his thigh, or on a table, and rubs it with the other hand, from the palm towards the finger tips, stretching the stiff joints into extension. A little oil helps, but is not essential.

The active exercise is done with the affected hand lying in the same position, but the ulnar border of the other hand is pressed firmly into the upturned palm. The patient then attempts to straighten the fingers of the lower hand. This exercise extends the interphalangeal joints, while preventing hyperextension at the metacarpophalangeal joints.

Following median nerve damage, the thumb web needs to be stretched: the patient grasps the distal end of the metacarpal bone of the affected thumb, and pulls it away from the fingers. Pressure must not be exerted on the phalanges as this will increase joint laxity.

Feet. For a person with foot drop, one passive exercise that helps to stretch the Achilles tendon is to stand erect, keeping the feet flat on the ground, and facing a wall about 70 cm away. With the palms of the hands flat against the wall, do 'press-ups' in the vertical position.

Eyes. First the patient should massage the skin over the orbicularis oculi muscles with the flats of the fingers, 30 times. Then, looking into a mirror, he should attempt to close the eyes as strongly as possible.

All these exercises can be carried out by a patient at home. If reconstructive surgery is to be performed, the patient will require more intensive preparation in a physiotherapy department.

Pre-operative physiotherapy

The aim is to teach the patient to identify the action of individual muscles. Many reconstructive operations require the patient to use a different muscle to substitute for the paralysed muscle. If the operation is to be a success the patient must learn to use that muscle in isolation from its synergists and antagonists *before* the operation is performed. It follows that the success of the operation depends upon the intelligent co-operation of the patient.

RECONSTRUCTIVE SURGERY IN LEPROSY

This account will not give detailed surgical techniques, nor prepare anyone to carry out the surgical procedures mentioned. Reference is made at the end of the chapter to excellent accounts of surgical techniques in leprosy which should be read by those intending to undertake surgical rehabilitation for leprosy patients. It should also be stressed that many of these procedures are only satisfactorily learned under apprenticeship, and must be supplemented by the pre- and post-operative assistance of a trained physiotherapist or physiotherapy technician trained specifically for leprosy.

The fact that surgery is indicated at all in leprosy is an admission of failure:

1. Failure to educate the public about the importance of early diagnosis and adequate therapy.
2. Failure in medical management of leprosy and its complications.
3. Failure to teach the patient how to live with anaesthesia.

The most frequently involved parts of man's anatomy in leprosy are also his most vital tools and his contacts with the world about him, i.e. his hands, his feet and his eyes. Every effort must be made to save these vital parts. There is little place for destructive or mutilating surgery. Digits and the bones of hands and feet should only be removed when irretrievably diseased and useless. If there is any question, take the road of conservatism and conservation. Then, teach and reteach the patient how to preserve his extremities.

Indications for reconstructive surgery

Reconstructive surgery that requires the intelligent pre- and post-operative co-operation of the patient should only be done if the patient is eager for help and is willing to co-operate.

If corticosteroids have been used within the previous 3 months they should be prescribed again for a few days over the time of operation.

Adequate time should be given for a definitive trial of medical treatment before considering surgery. Many paralysed muscles will regain function if proper therapy is given (see Ch. 8). Return of muscle function is common after radial paralysis and wrist drop. Muscles innervated by median and ulnar nerves less frequently regain function, but will sometimes do so within the first year of medical management of reactional states. Drop foot may improve up to 18 months after its onset or even longer. The younger a patient is, the better the prognosis. A patient beyond 40 years of age seldom regains lost function.

When muscle function recovers as a result of medical treatment and physiotherapy, the results are significantly better than those following the best reconstructive surgery.

The use of clofazimine, with its dual action in the management of reactions, has reduced the need for surgery and has allowed surgery to be offered earlier than was previously possible.

Surgical procedures can be divided into functional and cosmetic.

Procedures for improvement of function

Face

Surgery is the only treatment for entropion and trichiasis. Standard procedures are used in leprosy.

Two procedures are commonly used for lagophthalmos:

Tarsorrhaphy, or partial closure of the palpebral fissure (Fig. 12.6). This can be done laterally, medially or both, and may be temporary or permanent. Lateral tarsorrhaphy is the simplest and most effective. It is done by removing a strip of skin and conjunctiva on opposing lid margins at the lateral fornix and one third of the lower tarsal plate. The raw surfaces are sutured together to narrow the palpebral fissure. Medial tarsorrhaphy must be confined to the area medial to the puncta. The best result is obtained by doing a Z-plasty. Tarsorrhaphy disfigures only if unilateral. If bilateral it makes little noticeable difference in appearance.

Temporalis transfer. This is a more satisfactory procedure than tarsorrhaphy in that it provides active closure but unfortunately few patients have sufficient incentive to use it properly and it becomes simply a static sling. A slip of temporalis muscle is rerouted from above the zygoma toward the eye, and two extensions of temporalis fascia are led to encircle the eye and are fixed to the medial palpebral ligament. They are activated by the slip of muscle when the temporalis contracts. If lagophthalmos is complicated by corneal anaesthesia this procedure does not provide a good result as the patient receives no external stimulus to blink and he is unlikely to remember to do so. Tarsorrhaphy is then preferable.

Facial nerve palsy with inability to close the mouth. A static graft

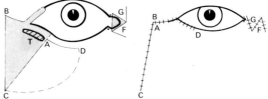

Fig. 12.6 Tarsorrhaphy of lagophthalmos of right eye.
Lateral tarsorrhaphy: the shaded triangle of skin, the lateral third of the lower
tarsal plate, and the mucocutaneous junction beneath the lashes of the lateral
third of the upper lid are removed. ACD is undercut, and A is sutured to B.
Medial tarsorrhaphy: two V-shaped flaps (F & G) are raised, the intervening skin
and mucous membrane are removed, and the flaps are interposed and sutured.
This procedure is called a Z-plasty. The puncta are spared.

of fascia lata or plantaris tendon can be used to support the lower lip.
It will keep the mouth closed and thus prevent loss of teeth due to
drying and secondary periodontal disease and is also of cosmetic value.

Hands

Paralysis of intrinsic muscles of the hand. For ulnar paralysis two
procedures are commonly used to activate flexion of the
metacarpophalangeal joints and extension of the interphalangeal
joints:

1. Intrinsic replacement, by using a radial wrist extensor as the
motor, and lengthening it with a free tendon graft from the palmaris or
plantaris muscles or with fascia lata. The grafted tendon follows the
line of action of the lumbrical muscles and is attached to a lateral band
of the dorsal expansion of the extensor tendon. This method is suitable
for a mobile, supple hand.

2. For a stiffer hand, one that needs considerable pre-operative
physiotherapy, the superficial flexor tendon of the middle or ring finger
is used. The tendon is split into four tails and inserted into the dorsal
expansions.

**For median nerve paralysis resulting in loss of opposition of the
thumb,** the superficial flexor tendon of the ring finger is rerouted to the
thumb. This procedure restores opposition.

Fixed flexion contractures of fingers. Arthrodesis is the best
procedure, usually of the proximal interphalangeal joints, and
occasionally of the distal joints.

Severe damage to all three nerves, ulnar, median and radial is rare,
which is fortunate because it is very disabling and there are few
muscles left to substitute for those paralysed. Wrist drop can usually
be corrected by three transfers:

1. Pronator teres tendon into the extensor carpi radialis brevis and longus tendons.
2. Flexor carpi radialis tendon into extensor digitorum communis tendon.
3. Palmaris tendon into flexor pollicis longus tendon. Later on, intrinsic replacement with superficial flexor tendons of ring and middle fingers for ulnar and median loss may be performed. Occasionally, however, arthrodesis of wrist or finger joints needs to be performed because of lack of adequate musculature.

Foot

Drop foot. This is the commonest deformity of the foot needing reconstructive surgery. The standard procedure is to transfer the tendon of the posterior tibial muscle to an insertion on the dorsum of the foot. Pre- and post-operative education is difficult and the operation should only be attempted when a physiotherapist with special training is available.

Tarsal bone disintegration. Treatment is slow and may be discouraging if a careful routine is not followed. The joint is immobilized in a walking plaster for 9 months. The plaster is removed for a very cautious trial of walking. Walking is gradually increased, with the support of an elastic bandage, and with periods of rest, so long as signs of inflammation do not return.

With mismanagement or lack of patient co-operation, the only option may be triple arthrodesis. In this complication of leprosy, more than any other, patience may be rewarding.

Dislocation or fixed deformity of the ankle is corrected by a wedge resection of the joint, fixing it in proper alignment to provide a plantigrade foot by the insertion of Steinman pins on each side of the resection, which are then pulled firmly together by external clamps and held until union has taken place.

Clawing of toes is commonly seen. It allows excessive pressure to be exerted on the metatarsal heads. For the great toe correction is provided by releasing the extensor hallucis longus from the distal phalanx and attaching it to the first metatarsal head and by arthrodesing the interphalangeal joints. For the other toes the long flexor tendons are transferred to the extensor expansions.

Amputation. When there is no feasible means of establishing a mechanically strong arch, as follows the total destruction of the talus or calcaneus, there is no alternative to amputation. Amputation is also indicated when malignant degeneration complicates prolonged ulceration. Some low-grade epitheliomas can be successfully excised and skin grafted if they do not involve deeper structures.

The stump should be as long as is possible, allowing for the end to be covered with a good layer of muscle or subcutaneous tissue. Amputation is usually carried out at the junction of the lower and middle thirds of the leg; but this site may be varied, for example if there is osteomyelitis of one of the long bones.

Cosmetic procedures

Cosmetic procedures are done for social and vocational reasons if the patient would otherwise be rejected by society or family or prevented from obtaining a job. These are very important in parts of Asia but not so important in Africa.

Face

Replacement of eyebrows. Hair transplants from scalp by free or pedicle graft.

Nasal collapse. Support of the nasal contours by a prosthesis or bone graft strut, after skin grafting to replace the destroyed mucosa.

Sagging face and ear lobes. Simple plastic procedures to remove excess skin.

Hands

In a few areas of the world the wasting or intrinsic atrophy of the hands is a stigma. Grafts of tissue or injections of foamed silicone rubber have been used to fill the defects.

Gynaecomastia

This embarrasses the patient and may be a stigma of leprosy. Simple mastectomy is performed through an incision which runs three-quarters of the way around the margin of the areola. A small piece of breast tissue is left immediately under the areola. This procedure is simple and gives a gratifying result.

Prosthetics

The commonest prosthesis required in leprosy is an artificial leg for a below knee amputation. The prosthesis should come into contact with and bear weight over as large a surface area of the stump as possible in order to minimize the risk of undue pressure at a particular point which will cause ulceration of an anaesthetic limb. Hence the value of a long, well covered, stump.

A technique has been developed for making below knee prostheses which is of use in situations where conventional prosthetic services are not available. It is suitable both for those who have leprosy, as well as for other amputees. The technique makes use of Plastazote as a liner; and the socket and body of the prosthesis are made of epoxy resins. The socket is made directly onto the patient's stump after the Plastazote has been moulded onto it. It is a total-contact socket similar to a conventional patellar tendon bearing socket. Making the prosthesis directly on the limb rather than on a plaster of paris model makes the procedure simpler, speedier and cheaper.

A rubber strap is made from the inner tube of a car tyre. The strap runs from the postero-medial brim of the socket, crosses the popliteal space, encircles the leg above the patella and recrosses the popliteal space to the postero-lateral brim. This provides adequate support but yet allows good mobility of the knee.

A foot is not added as it increases the cost, and is subject to rapid wear. Most patients find it easier to control a leg with a large round peg-like end.

FURTHER READING

Brand P 1966a Insensitive Feet. The Leprosy Mission, London
Brand P 1966b The hand in leprosy. In: Pulvertaft R G (ed) Clinical Surgery, vol 7. Butterworth, London, pp 279–295
Crenshaw A H (ed) 1971 Campbell's Operative Orthopaedics. C.V. Mosby, St. Louis
Fritschi E P 1984 Surgical reconstruction and rehabilitation in leprosy. The Leprosy Mission, New Delhi
Furness M A 1967 Physical therapy in the management of recent paralysis in leprosy. Leprosy Review 38: 193–196
Kaplan E B 1965 Functional and surgical anatomy of the hand. Lippincott, Philadelphia
Karat S, Furness M A 1968 Reconstructive surgery and rehabilitation in leprosy. Physiotherapy 54: 317–322
Kelly E D 1981 Physical therapy in leprosy for paramedicals — Levels I, II & III. American Leprosy Missions, Inc.
McDowell F, Enna C D 1974 Surgical Rehabilitation in Leprosy. Williams & Wilkins, Baltimore
Mendis M 1965 Physiotherapy in leprosy. John Wright & Sons, Bristol
Neville P J 1983 Footwear manual for leprosy control programmes, No. I & II, German Leprosy Relief Association, Würzburg
Neville P J, Rimondi R (eds) 1981 A simple sandal for insensitive feet. ALERT, Addis Ababa.

Soderberg T, Hallman G, Stenstrom S, Labo D, Pinto J, Marorf S, Velut C 1982
   Treatment of leprosy wounds with adhesive zinc tape. Leprosy Review 53: 271–276
Srinivasan H 1984 To care for leprosy as if the patient mattered. Indian Journal of
   Leprosy 56: 386–395
Tuck W H 1971 Problems in foot wear for the leprosy patient. International Journal of
   Leprosy 39: 633–639
Warren A G 1972 The management of tarsal bone disintegration. Leprosy Review,
   43: 137–147
Warren A G 1973 A study of the incidence and outcome of foot weakness in leprosy.
   Leprosy Review 44: 203–212

13. Social, psychological and vocational rehabilitation

Rehabilitation means the restoration of the patient to his former physical and social state so that he resumes his place in his home, his society and his work. To achieve this, treatment of the disease itself (Ch. 6) as well as the physical disability (Ch. 12) is necessary; but it must be accompanied by education of the patient, his family and the public, so that not only can he take his place, but also that society accepts him and assists him positively to do so.

STIGMA AND PREJUDICE

In many parts of the world leprosy still has a special position among diseases. There is, regrettably, a deeply entrenched prejudice against patients with leprosy which is more difficult to combat than that related to any other disease. No other disease causes such a reaction from the community and so much distress to the patient and his family. Sometimes the prejudice is more difficult to treat than the disease.

It is probably the extremely slow progression of leprosy and the amount of disability it causes that singles it out. *M. leprae* is a successful parasite that has established a balance with its host so that it thrives without killing him, while he becomes more and more grotesque to his fellow man. Most other disabling diseases would have killed the patient much earlier so that he would not be there as a reminder of the horrors the disease can produce. It is only natural for people to think 'I don't want to become like so-and-so who has been sitting begging by the wayside for untold years, blind and disabled'.

The functional disability caused by leprosy is often less of a problem than the deformity which disfigures and stigmatizes the patient. Unfortunately the average person fears the patient who looks grotesque although the disease process may be burnt out, while the patient who is infectious goes unnoticed, as the physical signs of leprosy are so slow to appear. For this reason isolation of leprosy patients is of little or no public health value, and only increases stigma.

In this respect the most significant thing we, as doctors, can do for the patient is to set an example in the community. It is easy to forget or overlook the fact that the lay community follows our example and attitudes towards patients and their diseases. Thus when we discuss education it is not only education of the patient and of the public that needs to be considered but, more important still, the education of medical workers so that they take a rational and helpful attitude toward leprosy patients.

AVOIDING THE NEED FOR REHABILITATION: OUTPATIENT CARE

There are many advantages of outpatient care. If the patient can be treated while he lives at home, he will never need to be restored to society. The patient is willing to start treatment at an early stage, long before he would agree to go off to hospital. Early treatment rapidly reduces infectivity so that transmission virtually ceases after a few days. In this way home treatment produces a 'chemical isolation'. The patient can continue his normal relationships and contacts and in most instances his normal occupation. He does not become estranged from his own society and will not need rehabilitation of any kind.

The problems of developing a workable system of outpatient care deserve all our effort and study. If outpatient treatment is widely available and accepted by patients much of the problem of leprosy is solved. But once a patient has been away from his family and familiar surroundings he becomes used to another situation, especially where there are others who have the same disease and disabilities. He joins the group — the 'tribe' or club of those with leprosy — and feels more at home with its members than with his blood relations.

Every effort must be made to keep hospital treatment to a minimum. The longer a patient stays away from home, the more difficult it is for him to return. After three years it may be impossible to return him to his original home.

There are many problems involved in the management of complicated leprosy, especially in situations where fear and prejudice are high, and it is easy to become emotionally over-involved and do too much for the patient. A delicate balance of firmness and love, of persuasion and education, is called for so that the patient's needs are met, but that he does not become dependent upon others, and wants to return to a life where he will have responsibility and self respect.

PROBLEMS OF REHABILITATION

Physical rehabilitation

The physical restoration of the individual to the best possible function is the first essential and is usually more easily attained than are the other aspects of rehabilitation. In some areas of Africa physical rehabilitation is of prime importance, for once that has been attained the person can return to normal life. Unfortunately this is not so the world over. In places where leprosy carries a marked stigma, the fact that a person is known to have had leprosy is sufficient to prevent his acceptance into society, even though there is no residual evidence of disease.

Psychological rehabilitation

In some communities, for example in parts of India and South America, the patient deliberately leaves his family in order to avoid the rejection of society which encompasses the rest of the family as well as the sick individual. Insurmountable problems may arise. He will probably lose his job, and without income his family is destitute. In addition he has the constant fear that he will transmit his disease to them. Then there is the concern that when he does recover, he still may not be accepted. He is plagued by fears, fear of being recognized as having leprosy, fear of rejection by his loved ones and fear of persecution by society.

A short period of hospital care at the onset of treatment has several points in its favour (see p. 90). In a society where the stigma is high, however, the patient accepts that he is an outcast and this attitude of mind is confirmed when he is admitted to a *leprosy* hospital. This should be avoided unless specialized care is essential. The problem will cease to exist when general hospitals are competent and willing to look after patients with leprosy.

The leprosy patient needs maximum psychological support. The family should be visited and reassured and its help solicited. In this way the education of the public as a whole is furthered.

Social rehabilitation

Education is the basic need. Educate the family and society to accept the patient as having simply a disease which is treatable and which is less contagious than most others they are familiar with. Educate them to accept responsibility for the patient in society and not in segregation, and for the dependants of the patient during the time he himself cannot provide for them. But society must not, out of fear, over-provide for the patient and ultimately deprive him of his self-respect and of his ability to care for himself and his dependants.

Legal measures

As the way in which leprosy is spread is not fully understood, it is impossible to say what are the most effective measures of control. Compulsory isolation has proved a failure. The provisions for control of infectious patients can and should be only those which are applied to any transmissible disease:

1. New cases should be reported.
2. Compulsory isolation and treatment should be considered only for infectious patients who refuse treatment.

No laws should be passed that apply solely to people with leprosy.

Management of leprosy in the general health services

One of the most effective measures to reduce the prejudice against leprosy patients is to provide for their everyday care in general medical units. Dispensaries, health centres and hospitals should be just as willing to accept and treat patients with leprosy as with any other infection. As with any disease that is a major cause of illness and that has peculiar problems there should be a specialist staff and facilities available for expert care of patients with problems that are beyond the routine knowledge of the average medical officer. But the ordinary treatment of leprosy and its more common complications and the education of the patient should be the responsibility of every medical facility. Not only does this make care more easily available, but most importantly it reduces the stigma of leprosy. Implementation of this policy will do more to gain acceptance of the patient into society than any other.

The role of voluntary organizations

Some patients with leprosy, especially those that are disabled, may need long-term assistance. Government hospitals in developing countries have very little provision for long-term patients. Medical staff are scarce and often uninterested in, or fearful of, leprosy. Regrettably, therefore, patients with leprosy are still largely cared for by missions and charities, a fact which in itself perpetuates stigma. Nevertheless long-term care of the severely disabled is likely to remain a suitable field of work for voluntary organizations, which should receive governmental assistance but retain full responsibility for their own administration.

A strong warning should, however, be given to avoid the risk of such aid increasing the dependence and loss of self-respect on the part of patients. Aid is only true aid when it allows the development of initiative and a desire to return to a normal place in society.

Assistance to patients' families

Where there is no other source of support, the patient's family, and especially the children, must be cared for by a welfare agency. But this should be only done as a last resort, when there are no relatives, friends or associates to shoulder the responsibility. It is best that such assistance be provided through agencies which care for similar needs for all sick people and not just those with leprosy.

Children of patients

The most humane, most economic and safest way to care for children of patients with leprosy is for them to live with their parents. To deprive an infant of breast-feeding is a death sentence in many parts of the world. Infants born of patients with leprosy should be protected with BCG and, when indicated, prophylactic chemotherapy (see p. 229). Children of patients with leprosy and children on treatment for leprosy should be regarded as normal and urged to attend the village school. Under no circumstances should special facilities for children of patients or child patients be provided. Children with multibacillary leprosy are not infectious after the first two days of an MDT regimen that contains rifampicin, and it is not necessary to take them away from school.

Experience in Nigeria over 15 years with over 1000 children living in close contact with patients has shown that, although some do develop leprosy, in no instance has it been severe nor has there been any disability or lasting evidence of disease. This is attributable both to the use of BCG and to the fact that the children have been brought early for diagnosis. The psychological, administrative and financial problems that arise from institutional care are thus prevented and the child has a relatively normal upbringing.

Cripples and beggars

These people are witness to the prejudices of society and the failings of the medical profession. In some communities the disfigured patient is accepted by society, but only as a beggar. In other communities begging is not socially acceptable and will not provide an adequate living. The latter situation is preferable, for when begging is discouraged the patient has to make himself responsible for his own sustenance. Where this is impossible he should be assisted by his family, or failing that, by the State or a welfare agency.

In an agricultural community in which leprosy is not stigmatized it is usually possible for patients to return to farming. Even with severe disabilities including blindness some are able to maintain themselves with little or no extra help. The attitude that this is the expected thing makes return to work practicable.

Vocational rehabilitation

Methods vary with the setting, with the attitudes of the people, with the opportunities for work for the able-bodied and for the disabled, and with the availability of farmland. In many situations the greatest hurdle is that of acceptance for employment of those who have or have had leprosy. Again, it is important to teach the community that these people can work, and are not going to spread the disease to others. There remain four factors that relate to the patient himself.

1. *He must learn to live with anaesthetic extremities:* to learn how he can work and yet not destroy his most valuable tools — his hands, feet and eyes.

2. *He must have the physical ability to work and have retained the initiative to do so.* This is not usually difficult in Africa. In other places such as North or South America and parts of India it may be practically impossible, due to lack of initiative and the prejudice shown towards leprosy patients by their fellow men.

3. *Training for a new job.* Some patients are so severely or selectively disabled that it is impossible for them to resume their old job, and retraining will be needed. Training should take into consideration the disabilities the patient has, including anaesthesia, so that in doing his work he does not increase his disability. It should also consider the opportunities in the society and other local social factors. It is no good training a person in a skill for which there is no opening, nor for a type of work that his caste or tribe forbids.

4. *Protected industries.* In only a very few situations is it practical and advisable to create protected industries specifically for leprosy patients. But if such industries exist for the employment of the disabled, they should be encouraged to take those disabled by leprosy.

EDUCATION

The most crucial factor in rehabilitation is education. Society needs to be educated to accept the person with leprosy. The patient himself must be educated in the importance of adequate treatment, and in how to protect his body from further damage. The example set by the medical profession in how they treat patients with leprosy and in the respect and consideration they show them as responsible individuals is of utmost importance.

FURTHER READING

Karat S 1968a Preventive rehabilitation in leprosy. Leprosy Review 39: 39–44
Karat S 1968b Preventive rehabilitation in leprosy, 3: principles of practical application. Leprosy Review 39: 75–8
Kaufmann A et al 1982 The social dimension of leprosy. ILEP, London
Leprosy Review 1972 43, No. 2: entire issue devoted to 'The stigma of leprosy'.
Neville P J 1980 A guide to health education in leprosy. German Leprosy Relief Association, Würzburg
Worth R M 1968 Is it safe to treat the lepromatous patient at home? A study of home exposure in Hong Kong. Leprosy Review 36: 296–302
Wright E M 1976 Leprosy villages — are they all outdated? A survey to two leprosy communities. Leprosy Review 47: 307–311

14. Experimental leprosy

Armauer Hansen discovered the leprosy bacillus in 1873, described it in 1874 and suggested that it caused leprosy. This was the first bacterium to be proposed as a cause of a human disease and his theory was not readily accepted. Bacteriology was in its infancy. The first proof of a bacterial agent of disease was Robert Koch's demonstration of the transmission of anthrax in sheep in 1876. In 1882 Koch isolated *M. tuberculosis* and showed that it was the causative agent of tuberculosis. Despite this good start the study of *M. leprae* has lagged far behind that of other microbial pathogens, including viruses, because it could not be grown on artificial medium.

This defect would not have been so serious if an experimental animal could have been found in which *M. leprae* would multiply. Culture of *M. leprae* in vivo was needed:

1. To obtain basic bacteriological data about viability, infectivity, growth, pathogenicity and sensitivity to antimicrobial drugs.

2. To establish an animal model of human leprosy in order to study host–parasite interaction and so obtain a better understanding of the pathology which underlies the extraordinary range of clinical patterns. The essential requirements of such a model are:

    a. It should imitate the disease seen in man.

    b. The organism should be the same as, or very closely related to, that causing the human disease.

    c. The animal should respond to the organism as closely as possible to the way in which man responds.

There are models of leprosy in mice, armadillos and primates, each serving different needs. The earliest information from animals, however, was from rats infected with *M. lepraemurium*.

Although *M. leprae* cannot be cultured in vitro, limited growth in defined liquid media or cell culture is now possible. These and the newer molecular biological techniques are also contributing to the explosion in knowledge of leprosy.

RAT LEPROSY: INFECTION WITH *M. LEPRAEMURIUM*

M. lepraemurium is morphologically similar to *M. leprae* and could not, until recently, be cultured in vitro. It is a natural pathogen of rats in which it produces a fatal systemic disease that is unlike human leprosy, but it has made an important contribution to the bacteriology of leprosy.

In 1958, J A McFadzean and R C Valentine noticed that dead organisms could be distinguished by electron microscopy from live organisms by the irregular density of their disorganized cytoplasm. Two years later R J W Rees and R C Valentine were able to show similar degenerate bacilli in human leprosy and to correlate this with the irregular beading which is seen in a proportion of organisms in slit skin smears.

They went on to show that, in rats treated with isoniazid, the proportion of solid staining (live) bacilli fell very much faster than did the total bacillary count, and that a later increase of solid staining forms showed the emergence of isoniazid resistant organisms. This work proved the relevance of the Morphological Index introduced by S G Browne (see p. 64) to assess progress in human leprosy, several years before it was possible to confirm that beaded *M. leprae* were dead (Fig. 14.1). These studies also prepared the ground for the objective assessment of chemotherapeutic trials.

MOUSE LEPROSY: INFECTION WITH *M. LEPRAE*

In 1960 Charles C Shepard in Atlanta, Georgia was able to show that

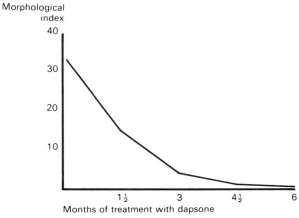

Fig. 14.1 Effect of treatment on the morphological index (after Rees, 1969).

M. leprae would multiply in the footpads of mice. Almost all our knowledge of the bacteriology of *M. leprae* and much information on the host-parasite relationship in leprosy comes from his work and that of R J W Rees in London.

Multiplication of M. leprae

An inoculation of 10^4 organisms will, after a lag phase of about 90 days, multiply logarithmically over a period of about six months to reach a plateau of about 2×10^6 organisms. Larger or smaller inocula produce the same final yields. This gives a generation time of 12 to 13 days during the phase of logarithmic growth, and an overall mean generation time of 18 to 42 days. After about 16 months the bacillary counts start to fall (Fig. 14.2). The optimal temperature for growth is 27–30°C.

The mouse footpad has been used as a culture medium to test the viability of *M. leprae* obtained from different sources and exposed to various adverse conditions. Thus, it has been shown that *M. leprae* in nasal discharges and in the blood of lepromatous patients are viable, that 10 years' treatment with dapsone or 2 years with rifampicin does

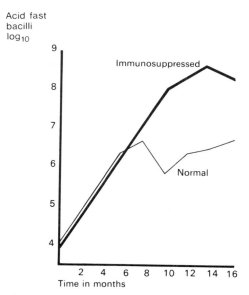

Fig. 14.2 Growth curves of *M. leprae* in normal mice and in mice submitted to thymectomy and irradiation with 900 R. After Rees (1969).

not kill all the bacilli in lepromatous patients, that smooth muscle, striated muscle and nerves are favoured sites in the body in which *M. leprae* can survive, that different drugs kill bacilli in patients at different rates (see Ch. 6), that very small doses of dapsone, while producing a good clinical response, consistently fail to kill bacilli in internal organs, and that *M. leprae* can survive outside the body for up to 2 days and occasionally longer. In nasal discharges, *M. leprae* survive up to 7 days in 44% humidity, or 14 days in 78% humidity. Mouse footpad inoculation is ten times more sensitive at detecting *M. leprae* than are slit skin smears.

Virulence and viability of different isolates of M. leprae

Many hundreds of isolates of *M. leprae* from all parts of the world and from patients with different types of disease ranging from LL to BT (it is not possible to isolate enough organisms from patients with TT) have been inoculated into mice. There is no evidence, so far, that different strains of organisms are responsible for LL or TT or that there are differences in behaviour between isolates from different parts. In mice, however, some strains reach their plateau sooner than others, produce higher total yields of bacilli and elicit less cellular response. These characteristics of fast and slow growing strains tend to breed true.

Proof of identity of M. leprae

The only certain way to identify an organism as *M. leprae* is to inoculate it into the footpads of mice, and to demonstrate its multiplication. Identity is confirmed by the histological character of the lesion in mice and by demonstrating the inability of the organism to multiply in standard culture media. Mouse footpad inoculation has been used to show that certain arthropods can take up *M. leprae* while feeding on lepromatous patients (see p. 206).

A much quicker and simpler screening test depends on the ability of *M. leprae*, unique among Mycobacteria, to oxidise dopa to melanin. A suspension of bacilli is mixed on a microscope slide and examined for change in colour.

Chemotherapeutic studies

The effect of drugs is tested on the logarithmic growth phase of *M.*

leprae. This has made it possible for the first time to assess the concentration of dapsone that inhibits *M. leprae*, to try new drugs in animals rather than in man, to distinguish between bactericidal and bacteristatic activity and to test for drug resistant strains.

Action of dapsone. In mice the minimal inhibitory concentration (MIC) of dapsone in serum is 0.003 mg per ml (see p. 78). This level is produced in man with a daily dose of 1 mg and human drug trials showed that such a dose was partially, but not completely, effective.

Trials of new drugs. Rifampicin was the first drug whose antileprosy activity was shown in an animal before being tried in patients. The success of this procedure meant that there was no longer any need to try new compounds in man without previous animal experiments and has enabled the testing of many hundreds of compounds among which ethionamide has been shown to be active.

Bactericidal or bacteristatic? Using a 'kinetic' method it is possible to distinguish between bactericidal and bacteristatic activity of drugs. The drug is given for only a limited period during the log growth phase. Bacterial counts are made from sample batches of mice at regular intervals and the time taken for bacterial growth to restart gives an indication of the mode of action of that drug. Rifampicin was shown to be bactericidal; dapsone, thiambutosine, clofazimine and streptomycin were bacteristatic. They failed to show any synergism between these drugs but did demonstrate antagonism against dapsone by isoniazid and para-aminosalicylic acid. `

Drug resistance. Resistance of *M. leprae* to dapsone had been suspected clinically for many years. This was confirmed in the mouse. Moreover it was found that the resistance ratio (MIC of dapsone for resistant strains/MIC for sensitive strains) was at least 100. Strains resistant to dapsone do not become sensitive again during passage in the mouse. A dose of 100 mg dapsone per day produces a therapeutic ratio (blood level/MIC) of 100. It is not yet known whether this has any effect on controlling the emergence of resistant mutants.

Immunization

Vaccination of mice with BCG significantly inhibits the multiplication of *M. leprae*. This is probably a result of specific immunity due to cross-reacting antigens, rather than the non-specific effect that BCG has in boosting cellular immunity. Dead *M. leprae*, or live *M. leprae* plus treatment, also protect mice, especially when given intradermally. Other species of *Mycobacteria* have proved ineffective.

Pattern of disease in normal mice

In the footpad of the mouse *M. leprae* multiplies preferentially in muscle cells and the cellular response is comparable to that seen in indeterminate leprosy in man. It was at first thought that, as the bacillary counts fell after 16 months, the infection died out. But if mice are examined histologically after two years pronounced changes are seen. Small numbers of bacilli are found in histiocytes and Schwann cells in dermal neurovascular bundles. There is also an epithelioid cell granuloma surrounded in places by loosely packed lymphocytes. This pattern is of borderline (BB) leprosy. Some bacilli were found to have disseminated to sites in uninoculated footpads and the nose, where bacillary multiplication was particularly prolific. The mimicry of human leprosy provides a model, the manipulation of which is rapidly increasing our understanding of the disease in man.

Pattern of disease in thymectomized, irradiated mice

It was not immediately apparent that infection with *M. leprae* in mice would, if left long enough, produce a disease like that in man, and it seemed likely that the tendency to recover was due to an efficient immune response. Attempts were therefore made to reduce the immunological competence of mice before infecting them, by thymectomizing them as adults and exposing them to sublethal irradiation with 900 R. This procedure destroys the cell mediated response and reduces the humoral response. In such mice:

1. *M. leprae* multiply at the same rate but reach greater final numbers of 10^9 bacilli (Fig. 14.2).
2. After intravenous inoculation lesions appear in nose, ears and feet and total bacillary counts are over 10^{10}.
3. Footpad inoculation is followed by early dissemination to these sites.
4. The histology of the lesions resembles that of lepromatous leprosy.

These findings confirm the suspicion that in man a deficiency of cellular immunity underlies the pathogenesis of lepromatous leprosy.

Leprosy in the nude mouse

In 1976 a mouse with no hair was discovered. This mutant also lacks a thymus gland, is deficient in T-cells, and is unable to mount a cell mediated immune response. The nude mouse is extremely sensitive to infection with *M. leprae*, and will detect as little as 100 live organisms among an inoculum of 10^8 dead organisms. Total bacterial counts reach 10^{10}, and there is a heavy infection of skin (especially of tail, ears and snout), testes, liver, spleen and lymph nodes. Bacilli are also present in endoneurim and perineurium, including Schwann cells, and in striated and smooth muscle and vascular endothelial cells.

Reactions

If thymectomized irradiated mice with LL leprosy are injected intravenously with syngeneic (genetically compatible) lymphocytes from normal mice there develops, ten days later, acute inflammation at the site of all pre-existing lesions. Clinically this resembles a type 1 reaction. Histologically, too: macrophages are seen to be degenerating, globi are broken open, lymphocytes are infiltrating the lesions and where they enter the perineurium the bacilli in Schwann cells are degenerated. This confirms that the pathogenesis of reactions accompanying reversal is a sudden increase in cellular immunity and hypersensitivity.

Transmission

In addition to the usual experimental route of inoculation which is subcutaneous or intradermal, leprosy can be transmitted to nude mice through the nasal mucosa, either by aerosols or direct application. Oral ingestion, pulmonary inoculation and bites of *Aedes aegypti* failed to transmit leprosy.

LEPROSY IN THE ARMADILLO

About 40% of nine-banded armadillos (*Dasypus novemcintus*, Fig. 14.3), inoculated with *M. leprae*, develop florid lepromatous leprosy, both clinically and histologically, after a year or more. There is enormous bacillary multiplication involving lungs and brain as well as other tissues more commonly invaded by *M. leprae*. The liver may contain as many as 10^9 bacilli per g of tissue. Such animals yield huge numbers of bacilli that can be used for metabolic and immunological studies. Most animals fail to develop the disease, but there is a tuberculoid response at the site of inoculation. The armadillo is susceptible to several other human pathogens, possibly because it has a low body temperature, 30–36°C, but little is known of its immune response.

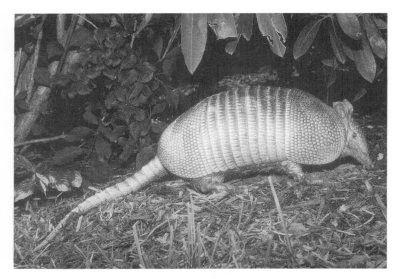

Fig. 14.3 *Dasypus novemcintus*, the nine-banded armadillo, which is particularly susceptible to infection with *M. leprae*, possibly because of its low body temperature.

Armadillos live for 12 to 15 years and produce sets of monozygous quadruplets, which could help in genetic studies of susceptibility, but the animal does not breed readily in captivity. Since 1975 increasing numbers of wild armadillos have been found with leprosy in Texas and Louisiana (see p. 204).

The smaller seven-banded armadillo (*Dasypus hybridus*) adapts better to captivity, breeds more readily and is easier to handle. It develops leprosy more quickly than the nine-banded, and could become a more useful experimental animal.

LEPROSY IN PRIMATES

The discovery of naturally acquired leprosy in a Mangabey monkey (*Cercocebur atys*), led to revival of interest in primate models of leprosy. Experimentally infected Mangabeys develop lepromatous leprosy and die after approximately four years. Skin, nasal mucosa, peripheral nerves and testes are heavily bacillated by *M. leprae*, but internal organs are little involved. Immunological studies show a T-lymphocyte defect similar to that found in man. Rhesus (*Macaca malatta*) and African green (*Cercopithecus aethiops*) monkeys are also under investigation as suitable and more convenient models.

MYOBACTERIUM LEPRAE IN CELL CULTURE AND SHORT-TERM MAINTENANCE IN VITRO

M. Leprae may be maintained alive in mouse or human macrophage cultures for several weeks, and also in certain complex media for a similar period. These bacteria are metabolically active, as demonstrated by uptake of radiolabelled thymidine. These systems are being tested for ability to demonstrate the effect of drugs, and the presence of dapsone resistance.

In vitro cultures of nerve tissue or of purified Schwann cells and neurofibroblasts, have been used to study the interaction of *M. leprae* with nerves. *M. leprae*, but not other *Mycobacteria*, adhere to the surface of Schwann cells, and are phagocytosed. Schwann cells and neurofibroblasts will phagocytose *M. leprae*. *M. leprae* will not invade the axon. *M. leprae* will multiply in Schwann cells. Affected Schwann cells do not associate in the normal way with axons, and do not synthesize myelin. Successful chemotherapy may restore Schwann cell function. *M. leprae* itself is not toxic to the cells in culture, but the addition of immune spleen cells induces cytopathic changes.

Attempts to culture *M. leprae* from man or armadillos in cell free media have often yielded *Mycobacteria* which, on critical evaluation, have proved to be another species. This has led some workers to suggest that the successful intracellular growth of *M. leprae* depends upon the presence of a second organism which supplies essential nutrients that *M. leprae* cannot synthesize. *M. leprae* has, however, been successfully maintained alive in liquid medium for 16 weeks, and been shown to multiply 2–3 generations before dying out. It has not been subcultured. This short-term maintenance culture has been used to demonstrate the efficacy of dapsone and rifampicin, and of some derivatives of trimethoprim.

MOLECULAR BIOLOGY OF *MYCOBACTERIUM LEPRAE*

The production of monoclonal antibodies and the application of recombinant DNA technology are two approaches which are proving useful in studying the mycobacteria.

Monoclonal antibodies are produced by fusing B-cells from mice, immunized with mycobacteria, with mouse myeloma cells, and plating the individual hybrids so that a clone of cells grows up secreting a single immunoglobulin, whose specificity is determined by screening against whole organisms or components thereof, or against antigens produced by an expression library (see below). These defined antibodies may then be used in mycobacterial taxonomy, diagnosis and epidemiology, and immunochemical detection of mycobacterial antigens. Monoclonal antibodies which react with lymphoid cells have proved useful in identifying cell types involved in leprosy granulomas (see p. 110).

Recombinant DNA technology is being used to produce and study *M. leprae* proteins. DNA, extracted chemically from *M. leprae*, is chopped into small pieces, either mechanically or using enzymes. These DNA pieces are inserted via a bacteriophage or plasmid vector into the DNA of *E. coli*, which is grown up in clones and will faithfully reproduce the inserted segment of DNA along with its own. In this way a genomic library is constructed, and the contents of the library — each clone with each segment of *M. leprae* DNA is likened to a single book — can be read by a variety of techniques. One such technique involves using single strands of DNA fragments which will bind or hybridize to their identical pairs. Alternatively antibody binding to expressed protein may also be used to read the library. Hybridization techniques may also be used to identify relatively small numbers of organisms — for example from soil or animals or insects. Theoretically, though in practice with difficulty, the *M. leprae* DNA in cloned *E. coli* may express its gene product — make the appropriate protein — in large quantities. These pure proteins may then be used in immunological studies that could, for example, lead to the production of a candidate vaccine. Enzymes of *M. leprae* expressed by the library could be used as targets for new candidate drugs. The potential of this technology has yet to be realized.

FURTHER READING

Dhople A M, Green K J 1988 Limited *in vitro* multiplication of *M. leprae*; application to screening potential anti-leprosy compounds. Health cooperation papers — 7, Nunzi E (ed). Associazione Italiana "Amici di R. Follereau", O.C.S.I, Bologna 23–31

Johnstone P A S 1987 The search for animal models of leprosy. International Journal of Leprosy 55: 535–547

Lancaster R D, McDougall A C, Hilson G R F, Colston M J 1984 Leprosy in the nude mouse. Experimental Cell Biology 52: 154–157

Mukherjee R, Antia N H 1985 Intracellular multiplication of leprosy-derived mycobacteria in Schwannn cells of dorsal foot ganglion cultures. Journal of Clinical Microbiology 21: 808–814

Nath I, Prasad H K, Sathish M, Sreevatsa, Desikan K V, Seshadri P S, Iyer C G S 1982 Rapid radiolabeled macrophage culture method for detection of dapsone-resistant *Mycobacterium leprae*. Antimicrobial Agents and Chemotherapy 21: 26–32

Rees R J W 1969 New prospects for the study of leprosy in the laboratory. Bulletin of the World Health Organization 40: 785–800

Rees R J W 1973 A century of progress in experimental leprosy. International Journal of Leprosy 41: 320–328

Seckl M J 1985 Monoclonal antibodies and recombinant DNA technology: present and future uses in leprosy and tuberculosis. International Journal of Leprosy 55: 618–640

Shepard C C 1971 The first decade in experimental leprosy. Bulletin of the World Health organization 44: 821–827

Storrs E E 1974 Growing points in leprosy research 1. The armadillo as an experimental model for the study of human leprosy. Leprosy Review 45: 8–14

Wolf R H, Gormus B J, Martin L M et al 1985 Experimental leprosy in three species of monkeys. Science 227: 529–531

15. Epidemiology

All the information on the epidemiology of leprosy would more than fill this book, but can be summed up in a sentence: the epidemiology of leprosy is still not fully understood — although the application of serology to epidemiology, and the development of the nude mouse model of leprosy have answered several questions about transmission and infectivity.

There are a great many difficulties in collecting and interpreting epidemiological data on leprosy. The most important are:

1. Patients are a self selected group and not representative of the population as a whole.

2. Studies of prevalence (proportion of population with disease at a given time) are easy to carry out but are retrospective and say nothing about transmission. Studies of incidence (proportion of population presenting with new disease each year) are difficult, expensive and time-consuming but much more informative.

3. Data are available from all over the world but the utmost caution needs to be exercised in interpolating them from one situation into another.

4. Leprosy spreads so slowly (see p. 1, 214) both in the individual and in the community that its pattern of evolution is seldom adequately studied.

5. Our inability to culture *M. leprae* in vitro deprives us of the most basic bacteriological information. This defect is being partially remedied by in vivo culture in the mouse and the armadillo (see Ch. 14).

6. Until recently there was no way of detecting subclinical cases, and those at risk of developing lepromatous disease (see below: *Who gets what type of leprosy?*)

This chapter presents information selected (a) in the belief that it is true and (b) in order to illustrate the difficulties encountered in studying epidemiology. It is intended as discussion, not dogma. The information is wherever possible qualified in order to prevent over-simplification and false deduction. The reader is invited to check the information at source and to draw his own conclusions.

The organism: *Mycobacterium leprae*

Aetiological agent

Leprosy bacilli are consistently found in cases of leprosy (in the range LL–BT); other pathogenic organisms are not. *M. leprae* produces a leprosy-like disease when inoculated into the footpads of mice (Rees 1969). Only one of many deliberate attempts to transmit leprosy in man has succeeded, and there are only four accounts of accidental transmission (Rees 1973, Wade 1948).

Reservoir

So far as is known man is the only natural reservoir of *M. leprae*. Experimental infections have with difficulty been established in hamsters, mice, some species of monkey and the nine-banded armadillo. 2–6% of wild armadillos in Texas and Loiuisana, though none so far in Florida, are infected with *M. leprae*. The infection is thought to have originated from man, but to spread among the armadillos. One infected armadillo may harbour up to 10^{12} *M. leprae*. Several armadillo handlers have caught leprosy (Lumpkin et al 1983, Storrs 1984). Four cases of leprosy have been reported since 1985 in Texas and Louisiana in people without known leprosy contact. Could the armadillo become an important reservoir of infection? (Job et al 1989). The role of clothing and of house dust as possible reservoirs is unknown.

One implication of this information, if correct, is that preventive measures need only be directed at man and the man–man cycle.

Multiplication, variability and viability

The generation time of *M. leprae*, during the logarithmic growth phase in mice, is 12–13 days, but different isolates show lag phases of different duration, so that the overall mean generation time from inoculation to plateau (see p. 193) is 18–42 days. Slow and fast growing strains, in this sense, breed true (Shepard & McRae 1970). This is, so far, the only difference that has been found between several hundred isolates from patients with leprosy in the range LL to BT from all over the world. The optimum temperature for growth in the footpad of the mouse is 27 to 30°C which is achieved with an ambient temperature of 20°C (Shepard 1965). If this holds for man why is leprosy so successful in the tropics where ambient temperatures are often over 30°C?

Boiling and autoclaving kill *M. leprae*. *M. leprae* in nasal mucus usually die outside the body within 2 days, but may survive up to 9 days (Davey & Rees 1974, Desikan 1977). Susceptibility to cold, water, drying, sunlight and disinfectants is unknown. They survive 0.5 N sodium hydroxide for 20 minutes, and in liquid nitrogen indefinitely. The natural lifespan of an individual organism in the body is not known, but live bacilli — persisters — can still be isolated from patients after 10 years of treatment with dapsone (Waters et al 1974).

Transmission

Source of infection

Who is infectious? Patients with lepromatous leprosy harbour most bacilli in their skin, but bacilli are seldom shed from intact skin: 20 out of 24 Nepalese patients with lepromatous leprosy had no bacilli on 813 cm^2 of facial skin surface. Twenty-five bacilli were found on the face of the other four, three of whom had a nasal discharge and one an ulcer (Pedley 1970). The nasal mucosa in lepromatous leprosy is heavily infected with *M. leprae* (Fig. 4.12, Plate 4), and the blood in subendothelial capillaries contains a greater concentration of bacilli, about 10^9/ml, than does peripheral venous blood. Bacilli are shed continuously through epithelial cells in mucus and in inflammatory exudate, or when the epithelium is injured or a capillary ruptures (McDougall, et al 1975). Nasal mucus contains *M. leprae* in 72% of LL, but in only 2% of BL, patients (Pedley 1973). The daily discharge of bacilli is of the order 10^7 to 10^8, and these bacilli are consistently viable (Davey & Rees 1974). Nasal secretions and lepromatous (as opposed to plantar) ulcers may be the main source of infection. Patients with tuberculoid leprosy have less bacilli but the cellular infiltrate reaches right up to the epidermis, which may ulcerate during reactions. At this time bacilli may be shed. There are, however, some epidemiological observations, such as the pattern of spread in an epidemic, which are not adequately explained by these hypotheses (Leiker 1960).

M. leprae may be found occasionally in the placentae of mothers with lepromatous leprosy. Although leprosy is very rare under the age of one year, babies of lepromatous mothers on treatment develop rising titres of IgM and IgA antibodies to *M. leprae*, showing that they have been infected. Duncan et al (1983) argue that infection is more likely to be transplacental than from nasal mucus or breast milk. Leprosy bacilli are found in breast milk of lepromatous mothers. Do they give leprosy to the child, induce immunity or induce immunological tolerance (see p. 94)?

Vectors

Blood of lepromatous patients contains viable bacilli in numbers great enough to be taken up by biting insects (Drutz et al 1974). Under experimental conditions, the mosquito *Culex fatigans*, and the bed bug *Cimex hemipterus*, can ingest *M. leprae* while feeding on lepromatous patients. Bacilli ingested by *Culex fatigens* have been shown, by mouse footpad inoculation, to survive up to two days (Narayanan et al 1972). Can these insects transmit *M. leprae* to man?

Tattooing has in several instances probably transmitted leprosy from man to man, and other cases of accidental transmission by intradermal injection are recorded. Must inoculation be intradermal?

Portal of entry

Apart from the few cases of accidental transmission the route by which *M. leprae* enters the body is unknown.

The first clinical lesion is almost always in the skin, and histologically bacilli are seen in the subepidermal zone or around pilosebaceous follicles. Alternatively there is lymphocytic infiltration of dermo-epidermal junction and the epidermis and bacilli are not seen. This is taken to represent maximum immunity to early infection (Ridley 1971). A report from India stated that one-third of child contacts had acid-fast bacilli in the skin without clinical signs of disease anywhere on the body (Chatterjee 1976). If they were *M. leprae* how did they get there? Down the hair follicle? Can they penetrate intact skin? Can they penetrate broken skin? It is said that in Asia where mothers carry babies on the hip that the first lesion is often on the buttocks, and that in Africa where the baby is carried on the back the first lesion is often on the forehead. But in fact such a baby turns its head to the side and the forehead seldom touches the back.

Single lesions of tuberculoid leprosy in India are distributed on exposed areas of skin. This distribution accords with clothing patterns of both sexes, and at different ages (Bedi et al 1975). Does this imply that *M. leprae* were inoculated intracutaneously at these sites, either by contact or by an insect? It has been suggested that the sharp spicules of palm frond matting may transmit *M. leprae* from one person to another.

The extraordinary infectivity of nasal mucus in lepromatous patients suggests that *M. leprae* may be disseminated by sneezing. Large heavy droplets fall to the ground where they might contaminate clothing or matting and be transmitted through the skin, or contaminate food and be ingested. Small, lighter droplets float as an aerosol which might enter the nose or eye or be inhaled into the lungs (Davey & Rees 1974). It is interesting that the rate of excretion of bacilli from patients with open pulmonary tuberculosis is similar, and that in India attack rates for the two diseases, analysed by age and sex, are roughly the same (Meade 1974). Do these observations suggest similar modes of transmission? Patients with early lepromatous leprosy commonly have nasal symptoms and the commonest site of lepromatous infiltration in the nose is the anterior aspect of the inferior turbinate bone, upon which inspired air first impinges (Barton 1974). This might suggest that the nose is a portal of entry or even site of inoculation. If so, why is the nose usually clear in BL leprosy? Do nasal lesions precede or follow dissemination in lepromatous leprosy?

Leprosy can be transmitted to thymectomized, irradiated mice by an aerosol of *M. leprae* (Rees & McDougall 1977). In nude mice (see p. 194) leprosy is transmitted if *M. leprae* are painted onto the intact nasal mucosa or inoculated subcutaneously, but not by painting them onto the skin, or inoculating them directly into the bronchi or stomach (Chehl et al 1985). Perhaps there may be more than one portal of entry into man, each of which is associated with a different immunological and clinical outcome.

Host

Who gets infected?

If *M. leprae* is transmitted primarily by sneeze aerosols, it would seem likely that all contacts of a lepromatous patient are liable to get infected, even if that contact is casual and brief. This hypothesis can be tested by the use of immunological tests.

Lymphocyte transformation (see p. 107) can be used as a test of specific cellular hypersensitivity. Using *M. leprae* as the test antigen, with BCG as the control antigen, a statistically significant relationship was demonstrated, in Ethiopia, between hypersensitivity and contact with leprosy (see Table 15.1). The results suggest that *M. leprae* may be more infectious than had previously been appreciated, and confirm the view that the great majority of people who become infected develop subclinical, immunizing infections (Godal & Negassi 1973). Tests of cell mediated immunity detect those who have been infected and have responded. Non-responders will be missed. This test may underestimate transmission.

No difference in positivity of lymphocyte transformation, however, was demonstrated between contacts of lepromatous and of tuberculoid patients (41% : 48%). Does this result suggest that tuber-

Table 15.1 Relationship between contact and infection in a leprosy endemic area, as shown by positive lymphocyte transformation to *M. leprae* (from Godal & Negassi 1973).

Nature of contact (numbers tested)	Percentage responders
None: under 2 months residence in Ethopia (26)	none
Residence in Ethopia over one year (45)	24%
Occupational contact with leprosy over one year (118)	53%
Ethiopian leprosy hospital staff office workers (12)	8%
workers in wards, physiotherapy etc. (27)	59%
workers in crowded outpatient department (17)	88%

culoid patients infect as many contacts as do lepromatous patients or could it suggest that contact with a lepromatous patient may be followed by reduced immunological responsiveness to *M. leprae*, or that many people are infected outside the house?

In Japan, Abe et al (1980) studied children in an area of low endemicity for leprosy, using a fluorescent antibody test (FLA-ABS) in which sera are absorbed with other mycobacteria to improve specificity (see Ch. 7). They found that 63% of all children and 92% of contacts were positive by the age of 5 years. This test is extremely sensitive, but is it as specific as claimed? Test sera from a non-endemic area were negative. Using a less sensitive, but possibly more specific test, the ELISA detecting phenolic glycolipid, it was shown in Sri Lanka that on average 34% of contacts were seropositive. Rates varied with the location, ranging from 10–55%. The highest rates were in children aged 10–14 years (Young & Buchanan, 1983). In India, 73% of contacts were FLA-ABS positive by the age of 5 years, compared with 33% of contacts of non-lepromatous cases (Bharadwaj et al 1982). If sero-positivity really is an indication of infection, these studies suggest that, in endemic areas, the great majority of the population is infected in early childhood, and that contacts of, especially, lepromatous individuals are at greatest risk of infection.

Who is susceptible to leprosy?

If this question could be answered in individual terms it might be possible by immunization, prophylaxis and surveillance to eradicate leprosy relatively easily and cheaply. The roles of genetic factors and acquired specific immunity are discussed on page 211.

Contact. In a community where leprosy is endemic, the risk of developing the disease is greatest among contacts of cases. For example, in an 8 year study in India, the attack rate among contacts was 6.8 per thousand, as compared with 0.8 per thousand without contact. The risk was doubled by multiple contact or by contact with a lepromatous patient (Rao et al 1975). The risk is increased by closeness and duration of contact. Thus, for patients in Louisiana who had a known contact, that contact was a parent in 100% of patients under 5 years of age, but in only 33% of patients over 10 years.

Even so about two-thirds of all patients have no known contact and there are individual records of patients who stayed in endemic areas for only short periods of time. How often is leprosy transmitted by a person whose infection is clinically inapparent?

In Ethiopia, 2 of 76 babies born to mothers with multibacillary leprosy on treatment developed leprosy within 17 months of birth (Duncan et al 1983). In Culion Leprosy Colony in the Philippines, before dapsone was discovered, 36% of babies left with their lepromatous mothers for 3–6 years developed leprosy before the age of 6. None of the children taken away from their mothers at birth developed the disease (Lara, 1961). The figures might suggest that intensity of infection lowers the age and increases the risk of the disease.

Age. Leprosy can occur at any age but is rare in infants (Brubaker et al 1985). Is this due to passively transferred immunity or to a long incubation period? Cord blood of babies born to lepromatous mothers contains IgG antibodies, and in one-third and one-half IgA and IgM antibodies to *M. leprae* (Duncan et al 1983). In Madras 20% of patients were under the age of 10 as compared with 3% in the southern USA. In Hawaii 45% were under the age of 20 as compared with 24% in the southern USA (Badger 1964). Is this simply a reflection of the fact that there is a greater incidence of leprosy in Madras and Hawaii than in southern USA? In families in Hawaii in which there were already cases of leprosy over half the new cases were under 15 years of age, but in previously uninfected families only one-fifth of the new cases were under 15 years. Does this suggest that opportunity of contact is the main factor in determining age incidence?

In endemic areas of India, age incidence rates show a bimodal distribution, peaking at 10–14 and 35–44 years (de Vries et al, 1985; Fig. 15.1). These data, taken with the sero-epidemiological data on the

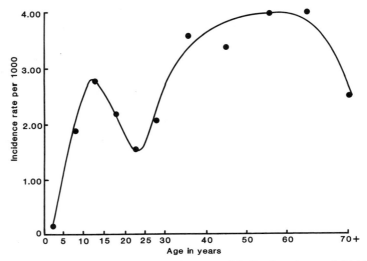

Fig. 15.1 Age specific incidence rates in a part of India where leprosy is highly endemic (from Nordeen 1985).

transmission of leprosy (see p. 208) suggest that leprosy in children is primary, and in adults mainly post-primary: not unlike the situation with endemic tuberculosis.

When leprosy dies out, as in Norway, Texas and parts of India, peak age incidence increases and the lepromatous ratio increases (Irgens 1985). Does this suggest that as social conditions improve, herd and individual immunity increase, and the disease is restricted to a few post-primary cases whose resistance breaks down as they get older?

Sex. In most prevalence studies males are affected rather more commonly than females. But males are more susceptible to lepromatous leprosy, and may be more forward in seeking treatment. In parts of Africa the male: female ratio is over 1 in hospital but under 1 at outpatient clinics. In Malaysia the male:female ratio in hospital is over 3:1. Sex differences are less noticeable in children and in epidemics. Are these differences related to opportunity of contact, clothing, hormones, genes or social factors?

Race. If frequency and severity of lepromatous leprosy are used as an index of susceptibility then white Caucasions are most susceptible, then Mongolians, then Indians, then Negroes. This pattern persists in emigrants. Does this also mean more susceptible to contract leprosy? What is the cause of the apparent relationship between skin colour and resistance to infection?

Acquired specific immunity. If leprosy is transmitted in early childhood, and adult leprosy is largely post-primary, what factors break down resistance and permit disease in adults (Bryceson 1981)? In one endemic area in the Congo, over an 8 year period, 25% of the population over the age of 20 developed leprosy (Browne 1974). With the exception of pregnancy (see p. 53), no responsible factors have been identified. The changing age pattern as leprosy wanes (see p. 210) suggests that the factors are environmental rather than inherited.

Immunity acquired from other mycobacterial infections. Infection with *M. tuberculosis* confers sensitivity to tuberculin. Tuberculin sensitivity does not of itself indicate any resistance to leprosy. Patients with leprosy appear to be fully susceptible to tuberculosis and vice versa. There is no good evidence of cross protection and yet BCG can protect against both. In Uganda BCG reduced the incidence of leprosy by over 80% in school children over a period of nearly nine years, but in Burma BCG was much less effective (see p. 223; Bechelli, et al 1973, Meade 1974, Stone & Brown 1973). This inequality in protection is even more striking when BCG is used against tuberculosis: 75% in Chicago, 31% in one part of Southern India, zero in another. One hypothesis is that previous exposure to environmental *Mycobacteria* preempts the way in which the body reacts to subsequent mycobacterial infection. Immunity may be so enhanced that the added effect of BCG is not detectable, or alternatively the immune response may be rendered inefficient, so that BCG is ineffective. If this hypothesis were proved, it might also account for some of the geographical differences in incidence and type of leprosy (Pallen 1984). The relationship between these organisms in terms of sensitivity and immunity is complex and conclusions should not be drawn hastily.

Who gets what type of leprosy?

Is there a genetic factor? Children and relatives of patients with leprosy do not get lepromatous leprosy more frequently than the population at large, nor does their type of leprosy concord with that of the contact (Horton & Povey 1966). If there is a genetic factor in susceptibility to leprosy it should be discernible in twins. Of 35 sets of twins in India in which leprosy was found, 23 sets were monozygotic (identical) and 12 were dizygotic. In 19 of the monozygotic sets both twins had leprosy and in 17 of them each twin had the same type of disease. In only 2 of the dizygotic pairs did both twins have leprosy and in neither case was it of the same kind (Ali & Ramanujam 1966).

These observations have been taken as evidence that there are certain people in every community who, if they get leprosy, are inherently liable to develop lepromatous disease, and that this liability is genetically determined (Newell 1966).

Genetic susceptibility to *M. lepraemurium* can be clearly demonstrated in inbred mice: C3H mice permit unrestricted growth of the organism while C57B mice develop a granulomatous response and contain the infection (Closs 1975). The gene responsible is within the H2 complex whose equivalent in man is the HLA system. It has proved more difficult to demonstrate HLA linked susceptibility to *M. leprae* in outbred man.

Studies of HLA frequencies in families with at least two affected and two unaffected children, have shown that children with tuberculoid leprosy share certain haplotypes more frequently than expected, notably DR2 and DR3 which are also more frequent in lepromin positive individuals and less frequent in lepromatous patients. Because lepromatous leprosy is relatively uncommon, HLA segregation may only be found in very large surveys. DQw1 is expressed more frequently in lepromatous patients and in lepromin negative individuals (Ottenhoff & de Vries 1987). These data suggest that genes affect the type of leprosy rather than susceptibility to the disease. How important is this genetic influence? Will it affect attempts at primary control (see p. 228)?

Prognostic value of lepromin. In a prospective study in India over 600 school children were tested with lepromin. Of those who were lepromin (Mitsuda) positive 3% eventually developed leprosy and in none was it lepromatous. Of those who were lepromin negative 15% developed leprosy and in three-quarters of them it was lepromatous. Lepromin negative children were retested three times and some of them converted to positive. Of those who failed to convert 62% developed leprosy and in five-sixths of them it was lepromatous (Dharmendra & Chatterjee 1956).

Does this suggest that lepromin (Mitsuda) negativity can be used as a prognostic index to identify people at risk? Lepromin (Mitsuda) positivity can be induced by natural exposure to *M. leprae*, by lepromin testing and by BCG inoculation, but in each instance there are people who fail to respond. There may well be other natural inducers of lepromin positivity. Patients with LL leprosy never become lepromin positive, even when healed. Is this inability to respond inherent in the host (genetic) or is it induced by *M. leprae* (acquired)?

Prognostic value of serology. Patients with lepromatous leprosy have higher titres of antibodies to more antigens than do patients with tuberculoid leprosy (see p. 110). Can individuals with subclinical 'pre-lepromatous' leprosy be distinguished from the majority of people with subclinical infections that will heal spontaneously? Ramu (1988) reported 17 FLA-ABS positive contacts whose sera were also positive in a monoclonal inhibition assay. Seven of them developed leprosy within one year as compared with 3 of 48 who were negative in the monoclonal test. In India, the FLA-ABS test was combined with lepromin testing in a study of 390 contacts. 1.5% of the lepromin positive/seronegative group got leprosy as compared with 14% of the lepromin negative/seropositive group (Ramu 1988). If these early results could be consistently repeated in other areas, might 'at risk' groups be identifiable for the purposes of control (Editorial, 1986)?

Leprosy as an imported disease

Leprosy is imported in immigrants into developed countries: 1700 into the USA in 10 years, 2000 into Great Britain in 30 years (Neill et al 1985). No secondary cases have been reported

Table 15.2 Differences in behaviour of leprosy in epidemic and endemic situations.

Epidemic	Endemic
1. The disease spreads rapidly. In Nauru in 1921 to 1925, 30% of the population caught leprosy.	The disease spreads slowly.
2. Cases are found in most villages and homes and no particular foci can be identified.	Cases are often clustered around foci of villages or families.
3. Most people get tuberculoid (BT–TT) disease which heals spontaneously.	*Relatively* more have lepromatous disease. There is a suggestion that 5–10 per 1000 of the population are prone to lepromatous disease in both situations.
4. All ages and sexes are equally susceptible.	Children and young adults are more commonly affected, and males more than females.
5. Contact with lepromatous patients does not seem to be important in determining the pattern of spread.	Contact with lepromatous patients greatly increases the risk of infection and affects the pattern of spread.

although lepromatous patients may not reach diagnosis for several years. What determines this remarkable herd immunity? Previous leprosy, BCG vaccination, living standards or some other factor? When leprosy is imported for the first time into other, less developed countries, epidemics are started.

Epidemic and endemic states

Epidemics may occur when leprosy is introduced into a population for the first time. After the epidemic has passed its peak the disease settles down into an endemic state. The behaviour of the disease tends to differ in the two situations (Table 15.2).

These generalizations bring home the dangers of generalization. Should one say leprosy is highly contagious or feebly contagious? Is contact dangerous? Are children especially susceptible?

And finally, could leprosy be eradicated before all the questions posed in this chapter are answered?

FURTHER READING

Abe M, Minagawa F, Yoshino Y, Ozawa T, Saikawa K, Saito T 1980 Fluorescent antibody absorption (FLA-ABS) test for detecting subclinical infection with *Mycobacterium leprae*. International Journal of Leprosy 48: 109–119

Ali P M, Ramanujam K 1966 Leprosy in twins. International Journal of Leprosy 34: 404–407

Badger L F 1964 Epidemiology. In: Cochrane R G, Davey T F (eds) Leprosy in theory and practice. Wright, Bristol, pp 69–97

Barton R P E 1974 A clinical study of the nose in lepromatous leprosy. Leprosy Review 45: 135–144

Bechelli L M, Gallego Garbajosa, Mg Mg Gyi, Wemura K et al 1973 BCG vaccination of children against leprosy: seven-year findings of the controlled WHO trial in Burma. Bulletin of the World Health Organization 48: 323–334

Bedi B M S, Narayanan E, Does A G, Kirchheimer W F, Balasubrahmanyan M 1975 Distribution of single lesions of tuberculoid leprosy. Leprosy in India 47: 15–18

Bharadwaj V P, Ramu G, Desikan K V 1982 A preliminary report on subclinical infection in leprosy. Leprosy in India 54: 220–227

Browne S G 1974 Self-healing leprosy: report on 2749 patients. Leprosy Review 45: 104–111

Brubaker M L, Myers M W, Bourland L 1985 Leprosy in children one year of age and under. International Journal of Leprosy 53: 517–523

Bryceson A 1981 The relative importance of specific immunity in protection against leprosy. Leprosy Review 52 (suppl): 93–108. (The whole volume is dedicated to the epidemiology of leprosy.)

Chatterjee B R 1976 Carrier state in leprosy. Leprosy in India 48: 643–644

Chehl S, Job C K, Hastings R C 1985 Transmission of leprosy in nude mice. American Journal of Tropical Medicine and Hygiene 34: 1161–1166

Closs O 1975 Experimental murine leprosy: growth of *Mycobacterium lepraemurium* in C3H and C57/BL mice after footpad inoculation. Infection and Immunity 12: 480–489

Davey T F, Rees R J W 1974 The nasal discharge in leprosy: clinical and bacteriological aspects. Leprosy Review 45: 121–134

Desikan K V 1977 Viability of *Mycobacterium leprae* outside the human body. Leprosy Review 48: 231–235

de Vries J L, Perry B H 1985 Leprosy case detection rates by age, sex and polar type under leprosy control conditions. American Journal of Epidemiology 121: 403–413

Dharmendra, Chatterjee K R 1956 Prognostic value of the lepromin test in contacts of leprosy cases. International Journal of Leprosy 24: 315–318

Doull J A 1962 The epidemiology of leprosy. Present status and problems. International Journal of Leprosy 30: 48–66

Drutz D J, O'Neill S M, Levy L 1974 Viability of blood borne *M. leprae*. Journal of infectious disease. 130: 288–292

Duncan M E, Melsom R, Pearson J M H, Menzel S, Barnetson R StC 1983 A clinical and immunological study of four babies of mothers with lepromatous leprosy, two of whom developed leprosy in infancy. International Journal of Leprosy 51: 7–17

Editorial 1986 Serological tests for leprosy. Lancet i: 533–535

Godal T, Negassi K 1973 Subclinical infection in leprosy. British Medical Journal 3: 557–559

Horton R J, Povey S 1966 Family studies in leprosy. International Journal of Leprosy 34: 408–416

Irgens L M 1985 Secular trends in leprosy: increase in age at onset associated with declining rates and long incubation periods. International Journal of Leprosy 53: 610–617

Job C K, Kahkoren M E, Jacobson R R, Hastings R C 1989 Single-lesion sub-polar leprosy and its possible mode of origin. International Journal of Leprosy 57: 12–19

Lara C B 1961 Leprosy in children: general considerations; initial and early stages. WPR/LEP/24, World Health Organisation, Geneva

Leiker D L 1960 Epidemiological and immunological surveys in Netherlands New Guinea. Leprosy Review 31: 167–168

Lumpkin L R III, Cox G F, Wolf J E Jr (1983) Leprosy in five armadillo handlers. Journal of American Academy of Dermatology 9: 899–903

McDougall A C, Rees R J W, Weddell A G M, Wajdi Kanan 1975 The histopathology of lepromatous leprosy in the nose. Journal of Pathology 115: 215–226

Meade T W 1974 Growing points in leprosy research. (2) Epidemiology. Leprosy Review 45: 15–21

Narayanan E, Shankara Manja K, Bedi B M S, Kirchheimer W F, Balasubrahmanyan M 1972 Arthropod feeding experiments in lepromatous leprosy. Leprosy Review 43: 188–193

Neill M A, Hightower A W, Broome C V 1985 Leprosy in the United States. Journal of Infectious Diseases 152: 1064–1069

Newell K W 1966 An epidemiologist's view of leprosy. Bulletin of the World Health Organization 34: 827–857

Nordeen S K 1985 The epidemiology of leprosy. In: Hastings R C (ed) Leprosy. Churchill Livingstone, Edinburgh pp 15–30

Ottenhoff T H M, de Vries R R P 1987 HLA Class II immune response and suppression genes in leprosy. International Journal of Leprosy 55: 521–534

Pallen M J 1984 The immunological and epidemiological significance of environmental mycobacteria on leprosy and tuberculosis control. International Journal of Leprosy 52: 231–245

Pedley J C 1970 Summary of results of a search of the skin surface for *Mycobacterium leprae*. Leprosy Review 41: 167–168

Pedley J C 1973 The nasal mucus in leprosy. Leprosy Review 44: 33–35

Ramu G 1988 Assessment of the risk of developing leprosy among contacts. Health

Cooperation papers — 7 Nunzi E (ed). Bologna; Associazione Italiana 'Amici di R. Follereau', O.C.S.I., pp 93–99

Rao P S S, Karat A B A, Kaliaperumal V G, Karat S 1975 Transmission of leprosy within households. International Journal of Leprosy 43: 45–54

Rees R J W 1969 Human leprosy in normal mice. British Medical Journal 3: 216–217

Rees R J W 1973 A century of progress in experimental leprosy. International Journal of Leprosy 41: 320–328

Rees R J W, McDougall A C 1977 Airborne infection with *Mycobacterium leprae* in mice. Journal of Medical Microbiology 10: 63–68

Ridley D S 1971 Pathology and bacteriology of early lesions in leprosy. International Journal of Leprosy 39: 216–224

Shepard C C 1965 Temperature optimum of *M. leprae* in mice. Journal of Bacteriology 90: 1271–1275

Shepard C C, McCrae D H 1970 A characteristic that varies between strains of *Mycobacterium leprae*. International Journal of Leprosy 38: 342

Stone M M, Brown J A K 1973 A trial of BCG vaccination against leprosy in Uganda. In: Abstracts of Tenth International Congress of Leprosy, Bergen.

Storrs E E 1984 Leprosy in wild armadillos. International Journal of Leprosy 52: 254

Wade H W 1948 The Michigan inoculation cases. International Journal of Leprosy 16: 465–475

Waters M F R, Rees R J W, McDougall A C, Weddell A G M 1974 Ten years of dapsone in lepromatous leprosy: clinical bacteriological and histological assessment, and the finding of viable bacilli. Leprosy Review 45: 288–298

WHO 1985 Epidemiology of leprosy in relation to control. Report of a study group. Technical Report Series 716, World Health Organisation, Geneva

Worth R M, Bomgaars M R 1982 Immigration and leprosy in Hawaii, 1960–1981. International Journal of Leprosy 50: 335–341

Young D B, Buchanan T M 1983 A serologic test for leprosy with a glycolipid specific for *Mycobacterium leprae*. Science, 221: 1057–1059

16. Leprosy control

THE PROBLEM

The World Health Organization estimates that there are more than 2000 million people living in areas with a prevalence of leprosy of at least 5 per 10 000 and who are therefore at risk of infection. It considers that one million new patients may be expected during a five year period, and that only 5.3 million of the estimated world total of 11.5 million patients have ever had any treatment. The problem before us is overwhelming, especially in that it relates chiefly to developing countries with few funds to spend on preventive medical programmes.

The main reason for control of leprosy is the prevention of disability. In India an outpatient control programme reduced the number of newly disabled people by 60% over a period of 10 years.

Ever since the discovery that dapsone inhibits the growth of *M. leprae*, it has been presumed that control of leprosy in a given community or geographic area should be feasible, and that with persistence we can eventually halt and even eradicate the disease. Infected individuals are thought to be the only source of leprosy bacilli — except for some wild armadillos in the southern USA — and if a high enough proportion of patients are adequately treated it is logical to assume that leprosy will eventually die out. The lowest prevalence rate at which transmission can still continue is not known but appears to be under 5 per 10 000.

Since the introduction of control projects, which mostly began with the widespread adoption of treatment with dapsone between 1947 and 1950 and continues with multidrug therapy, the stress has been on early diagnosis and treatment of established infections. This has been called *secondary prevention*. A statistical model developed for the World Health Organization suggests that this approach is not entirely effective, and that unless some new weapons are introduced into the control armamentarium, eradication will not be achieved in less than 200 years.

MEANS OF CONTROL

Historical

There was an epidemic of leprosy in Northern Europe in the Middle Ages. After a period of 300 to 400 years it waned and by the 19th century was of insignificant proportions. At that time there was no effective therapeutic agent, and it is often stated that the disappearance of the disease was due to the practice of isolation. But there is evidence that leprosy was declining before segregation was started, and there was never more than a small fraction of the patients segregated at any one time; and as lepromatous patients are often infective for years before signs of disease develop, it seems unlikely that isolation can have had much effect. Furthermore, many other changes were taking place in man's way of life, and it is likely that one or some of these were more significant factors.

Many Scandinavians took leprosy with them when they emigrated to the United States of America in the 19th century; but by the third generation it had died out. On the other hand the French, who settled in Nova Scotia and then as a result of persecution left and resettled in Louisiana, maintain a small residual focus of the disease, still the source of a few new patients annually. These people are rural, educationally backward, and have a low standard of living. Leprosy also persists in other ethnic groups in the USA, many of whom have a recent history of having come from an area where leprosy is endemic, but they also tend to live in relatively unsanitary conditions and have a low standard of living. As long ago as 1895 Armauer Hansen said that personal and household cleanliness would prevent the spread of infection and control leprosy. In countries where leprosy is presently endemic, it may be that general measures which improve the standard of living will prove to be as important in the eradication of leprosy as those taken specifically to control the disease.

Present approach

The biological balance between man and the leprosy bacillus is at present more or less equal and any partially successful measure, if well directed, should result in the decline of the disease.

Isolation is neither effective nor practical. It cannot be practised without cruelty and it encourages continued spread of disease from subclinical and hidden cases. It is expensive and perpetuates fear of leprosy. Dapsone alone rapidly produces a 'chemical isolation' (see p. 184). Any regimen that contains rifampicin makes the patient non-infectious within two days. Isolation is unnecessary.

Control of leprosy is at present based upon two principles: treatment of infectious cases and increasing the resistance of those at risk.

Treatment of infectious cases

Early diagnosis. Leprosy is defined as hyperendemic where there is a prevalence of over 10:1000, and as an 'important health problem' at 1:1000. In a hyperendemic area one method of initiating a programme of control is a leprosy survey. This is expensive but defines the size of the problem and finds a worthwhile number of cases. The most useful function of a survey is to teach the population the signs of early leprosy, explain that it is curable and tell them where treatment may be sought. A good educational campaign is the best way to enrol new cases. The examination of contacts of infectious cases is often more rewarding than a mass survey and should be continued for five years.

Mass surveys of populations or of selected groups such as army, police, labour gangs, urban slums and especially schoolchildren, should be used to look for several diseases at the same time, to immunize against the important local infections and possibly to treat simple ailments. A rough estimate of the prevalence can be determined by examining all school-age children. The total prevalence will be about 4 times the number of cases found (Fig. 16.1).

Early treatment, monitoring, case holding and compliance. The greatest problem is to persuade a patient who feels well and has no signs to go on taking medicine (*compliance*). Leprosy is not a painful or disabling disease until late in its course, and the early manifestations are often inadequate to persuade the patient to continue to attend the clinic (*case holding*). If it is left to the initiative of patients to present themselves for treatment, fewer early cases are found but case holding is much better. Young males are the worst offenders. They do not like to acknowledge sickness and often find clinic times impossible to attend. Distant clinics and prolonged treatment regimes, as with dapsone monotherapy, breed defaulters. Education, cooperation, short simple regimens and the optimism generated by MDT improve compliance and case holding. Patients who default must be visited at home and persuaded to reattend. Health staff themselves may fail to see the need and become indifferent.

A simple urine 'spot' test that develops a colour on paper is available to detect dapsone in urine; the test is positive if dapsone has been taken within the previous three days. MDT drugs may be dispensed in

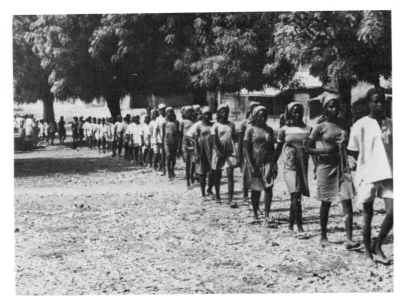

Fig. 16.1 In good time! Examination of all schoolchildren will give a good idea of the leprosy problem in any area. They are likely to contain a quarter of all cases and a higher proportion of new cases. Early diagnosis and treatment will prevent deformity and save individual suffering, reduce the burden on the community and help to eliminate the stigma of the disease.

'blister' calendar packs, in which each day's medication is separately laid out on a card and clearly labelled. Each month the previous pack is examined at the clinic for compliance, and a new pack issued (Plates 3, 6 and 7; Fig. 16.2).

It has been estimated by the World Health Organization that if 75% of infectious cases attended for treatment 75% of the time, transmission would eventually cease. Nowhere has this yet been achieved. One major difficulty is to define the early infectious case.

Outpatient care. Clinics must be set up within reach of the patients. They can be at hospitals or health centres or at a convenient meeting place, attended weekly by a dispenser. In some situations mobile clinics are useful but are much more expensive to run and tend to be less reliable. Every effort should be made to make clinics as convenient as possible for the patients in place and time. Holding the clinic on market day is an added incentive to come.

A register is kept at each clinic with the patient's name and address and each attendance or absence is recorded.

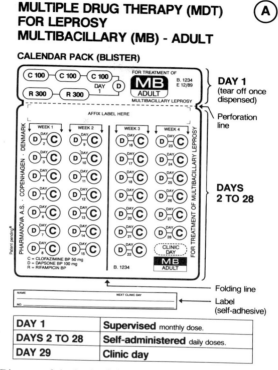

Fig. 16.2 Diagram of the back of the pack for multibacillary leprosy. The pack for paucibacillary leprosy is smaller and simpler in design.

The clinic should be visited regularly by a doctor to encourage the dispenser or attendant, check on treatment, look for cases in need of hospital care and discharge patients who are cured. Patients should realize that the clinic is for their benefit. If it is not managed properly they have a right and duty to report the matter.

Education — the key to success. The objective should be to evoke in the community, the patient and his family a reasonable attitude towards leprosy which neither exaggerates the danger of infection nor yet minimizes it. Full use should be made of all techniques of health education. Educate the public to recognize early leprosy and to understand that it can be successfully treated. Educate the patients where to go for treatment. Teach them the necessity of attending regularly. Assist the disabled to get medicine. Educate staff to be sympathetic and encouraging to patients. Teach them the need to look for patients who fail to attend and to find out why because ignorance, disinterest or disability often underlie irregular attendance, especially in young males with TT and BT disease. Another high risk group is females of marriageable age, who are likely to move to another area.

Prevention of disability and rehabilitation. This does so much for morale that new patients are encouraged to come. As the number of crippled and disfigured diminishes the public loses its fear and prejudice, and leprosy its stigma. Clinic staff should be taught to assess and record nerve tenderness and motor and sensory function regularly. They should know when to refer patients for reactions or protective footwear, and in an emergency be able to dispense corticosteroids to cover the patient's trip to hospital.

Training and administration. Without adequate trained staff and a sound administration no health programme can succeed. Important factors to consider in planning a programme are:

1. The size and nature of the problem to be tackled.
2. The staff already available, and the staff potentially available for training.
3. The resources of funds and facilities to be allocated, and for how long.
4. The cooperation of existing health services and staff, and how to make most use of them.

Implementation of multidrug therapy. It is possible to establish MDT regimens and MDT based control schemes in most areas, although in some remote places scattered population, lack of public transport, and natural hazards such as drought may make them impracticable. But planning, effort and care are needed for success. An initial survey is useful to define or redefine the problem. Questions that need to be answered include:

1. What is the extent of the clinical problem?
2. What is essential for the scheme to start? Increased staff, staff training, supplies, drugs, transport, better laboratory facilities and techniques, accurate records, money? Many of the old methods and attitudes will need to be changed.
3. Which patients should be included, excluded?
4. How to educate patients and the community, before and during the campaign.
5. How to monitor drug intake.
6. Pilot studies in one or two rural and urban areas help iron out unforeseen problems.

7. Targets for numbers and time must be defined and a policy for managing reactions instituted.
8. Evaluation of progress.
9. As the number of registered cases falls after the first few years, staff must be retrained to manage disability, search for new cases, insist on good follow-up rates and even use their experience to take on the control of other diseases, such as tuberculosis. Viewed in this way, the investment in MDT will more than pay for the initial increase in costs.
10. Finance. The cost of drugs for MDT, bought in bulk, and shipped to a developing country, is of the order of $6 for six months treatment per paucibacillary patient, and $26 for two years per multibacillary patient (in 1986). This represents 10–20% of the total cost of the programme.

Integration of leprosy conrol into the general health service. Historically the control of leprosy, like small-pox and yaws, has in some countries preceded the development of a general rural health service. The introduction of dapsone made it possible to develop a mass antileprosy campaign before the establishment of basic health services. But leprosy control should now be integrated into the general health service and this should be done at a time when:

1. The incidence has been reduced to an acceptable level.
2. The general health service covers the country widely enough and is adequately supported by government.
3. Adequate medical, nursing and primary health care staff are available, and have been educated in diagnosis and treatment of leprosy.

Increasing resistance of those at risk

In an epidemic up to 30% of the population may eventually become infected, but under 2% get lepromatous disease. In a hyperendemic area the prevalence of leprosy is usually well under 5%. The population at risk in a community is therefore usually small. At the moment there is no practical means of identifying this population and protecting it, and all those exposed to infection need to be protected alike.

Immunization. There is no specific vaccine for leprosy. Trials of immunization with BCG have been carried out in large numbers of children in Uganda, where it provided, overall, about 80% protection, and in Malawi and New Guinea about 50%. The level of protection varied markedly with age. In Burma, BCG gave 40% protection to those under 5 years of age; older children were not protected. Protection was only against tuberculoid disease. Virtually no information on protection against lepromatous disease is available. From these figures it is difficult to assess the value of BCG. It is possible that the differences between Uganda and Burma may be racially determined. BCG should be given for its value in preventing tuberculosis, but to give optimum protection against leprosy it should be given during the first year of life.

Vaccination trials are in hand using heat killed *M. leprae* combined with BCG, and with other species of *Mycobacteria*.

Prophylactic chemotherapy. Mass prophylaxis with oral dapsone is impracticable and might be expected to encourage the emergence of resistant strains. In Micronesia, a repository injection of acedapsone (DADDS) was given every 75 days to the whole Pingelapese population over the age of six months for a period of three years. After one year the incidence of leprosy fell from 25 per 1000 to zero. No new cases were seen while acedapsone was continued, but within a year of stopping prophylaxis, new cases, which were mainly lepromatous, appeared. In another study in India, acedapsone given every ten weeks for three and a half years afforded nearly 50% protection to child contacts of lepromatous patients. This approach might be applicable in geographically well defined areas, but must be followed by careful surveillance aimed at detecting the early lepromatous case whose disease had been temporarily suppressed by acedapsone.

Chemoprophylaxis is recommended for children under the age of 10 years, whose parents or household contacts are infectious (LL/BL, discharging bacilli from the nose or with a morphological index over 1%) and are receiving regular treatment. Prophylactic dapsone given in full doses (see p. 79), for three years offers about 50% protection. Six months chemotherapy with dapsone and rifampicin, as for paucibacillary leprosy (see p. 86) should offer even greater protection. Older children, or children of non-infectious parents, do not benefit. A baby at the breast of a mother taking dapsone receives adequate protection until weaning.

EFFECTIVENESS OF CONTROL MEASURES

Results

In several countries no effective programme of leprosy control has been established because of lack of funds, staff, facilities, or initiative. In others, varying degrees of control have been attained.

So much depends upon the social attitudes and prejudices of people against leprosy that these are often the basic factors in determining the effectiveness of the programme. It is all too common to find that the stigma is greater in the upper socio-economic groups and patients will refuse to come for treatment if it is offered in a setting that is known to be specifically for the treatment of leprosy. India is an example of a country where stigma has impeded some control programmes.

In Africa social pressures are such that regular attendance is more likely and control is easier. One reason for this is that people may come for the wrong reason. For example in some parts of Nigeria there is a belief that dapsone increases fertility. Where this belief is held, an entire village may come voluntarily for examination. All want to receive the 'miracle pill' and those elected to get it are the favoured few and they guard their right to it carefully, come regularly and take religiously every precious tablet. In this situation five years has proved adequate to get all those with leprosy on treatment and after a further seven years the incidence is very low.

In Tanzania, however, it has proved difficult to get more than 50% of cases on regular treatment. In Uganda, where control has been practised for 20 years, the incidence has more than halved in the last 10 years. But nowhere has leprosy been eradicated. The effect of control measures on the prevalence and incidence of leprosy in Japan is shown in Figures 16.3 and 16.4.

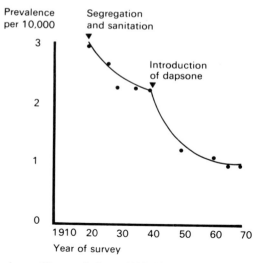

Fig. 16.3 Prevalence of leprosy in Japan 1919–1968, showing the apparent effects of segregation and sanitation, and of dapsone (from Yoshio Yoshe, 1970).

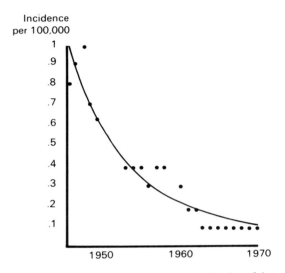

Fig. 16.4 Incidence of leprosy in Japan since the introduction of dapsone. Conventional control measures reduce incidence to a low level, but fail to eradicate the disease (from Yoshio Yoshe, 1970).

In spite of all the operational difficulties faced, several countries or projects have experienced a well documented decline of incidence during the last decades. Multidrug therapy is expected to accelerate that trend. In many countries where MDT has been widely introduced, a fall in prevalence by as much as 75% over five years has often been observed.

Results may also be measured by fall in the disability rate. With a successful campaign this rate falls by one-third in 4 years and two-thirds in 10 years. The rate with MDT is the same as with monotherapy, but the rate of recovery of lost function is much greater, rising from 20% to 50% in Malawi.

Finally, as control is achieved, the peak age of onset rises to about 25 years in males and 60 in females, and the new cases are predominantly lepromatous. These features imply that transmission has ceased and that the only cases are post-primary whose resistance cannot contain the infection acquired in childhood (see p. 209).

Problems

Time. Control of leprosy takes many years. In this time initiative declines and supervision becomes less keen. Although incidence decreases hospital facilities continue to be needed for care of complicated cases. The severely disabled have to be looked after indefinitely. As a means of control, MDT has dramatically reduced the duration of treatment of individual patients, reduced the numbers of patients that continue to attend clinics, and boosted the morale and efficiency of staff and patients. It remains to be seen whether MDT will make incidence rates fall any faster. This will determine how long the scheme has to remain in operation.

Terrain. A notable failure of control is seen in migrant peoples, such as the Fulani cattle herders of Northern Nigeria, who are always on the move to new grazing. No successful means of providing treatment has been devised and only a few with very severe disease or disability are willing to dislocate themselves from their way of life to settle in a place where they can continue regular treatment. Another problem area is in the slums of large cities, such as Bombay, where most of the patients are labourers. Many live on the work site and are impossible to trace.

Money. Leprosy is never headline news (cf. cholera, famine and drought) and it attracts little government money, especially when it is realized for how long funds must be committed. Annual budgets make successful planning impossible. Funds are usually insufficient to employ or train enough staff.

Staff. People brought up in a society where leprosy has a stigma do not want to work with leprosy patients. All too often staff lose interest because pay is inadequate and supervision lackadaisical. Leprosy attendants who have no medicines other than dapsone and whose only options are to give or to withhold it, are unable to deal with complications. The results are sometimes discouraging, and patients lose confidence.

Integration. When a leprosy service is integrated with the general health service it tends to take a secondary role and loses staff and funds.

Attitudes. The effect of attitudes of patients and public to leprosy control has been discussed above. Governments fail to realize that leprosy is one of the major disabling diseases in the country, and as such is of economic importance.

THE FUTURE

At present leprosy control means *secondary prevention*, or the detection and treatment of established disease. This has been practised now in some places for over 35 years, and it is evident that it is not eradicating the disease. Almost without exception the prevalence of leprosy has been significantly reduced world-wide, but whether this is due to all the effort and expense expended on leprosy control, or to the same factor or factors which led to the disappearance of leprosy from northern Europe in the last century, is unknown.

More fundamental approaches are needed in order to prevent the development of clinical disease altogether, by detecting individuals at risk and protecting them. This approach aims at what is termed *primary prevention*. Determination of the prevalence in leprosy is simple but ignores the time factor. Only with a study of incidence can we gain worthwhile information on the pattern of leprosy in the community that may help towards control. From incidence figures it

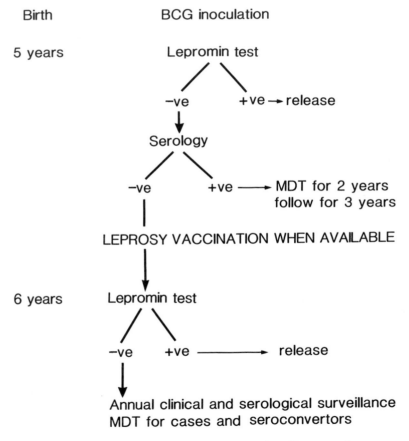

Fig. 16.5   One possible approach to primary prevention of leprosy, using immunological markers of susceptibility.

may be possible to determine high-risk factors and high-risk groups of individuals (see p. 207). Then it may be possible to prevent these factors applying, and to protect the groups from exposure. Contributory factors that still need study include age, sex, ethnic group, social and economic conditions. These must be carefully correlated in order to find out their effect on the development of disease. It is important that studies be done urgently, yet ethical considerations must not be ignored.

Another approach to primary prevention is to attempt to identify individuals at risk through genetic or immunologic markers. Genetic markers of susceptibility to lepromatous disease have not yet been identified in adequate detail to be of practical use (see p. 211). Immunologic markers are however available (see p. 106), although their theoretical powers of discrimination have not yet been adequately tested in the field. It would not be difficult to devise and test a scheme like that illustrated in Figure 16.5, to identify and monitor susceptible children, and to identify and treat early lepromatous cases, before they become clinically and bacteriologically positive.

Imaginative approaches will be needed if leprosy is to be controlled, let alone eradicated. The problem will become much more difficult, especially in Africa, if leprosy becomes an AIDS disease (see p. 106).

FURTHER READING

African Medical and Research Foundation 1977 A guide to leprosy control for field staff. ALERT, Nairobi

Brown J A, Kinnear Stone M M, Sutherland I 1969 Trial of BCG vaccination against leprosy in Uganda. Leprosy Review 40: 3–7

Buchmann N 1978 Leprosy control services as an integral part of primary health care programmes in developing countries. German Leprosy Relief Association, Würzburg

Collier P J 1983 A study of case holding in leprosy patients in Asia, based on duration of treatment, 1976–1980. Leprosy Review 54: 89–94

Convit J et al 1983 Immunotherapy and immunoprophylaxis of leprosy. Leprosy Review special issue: 47S–60S

Daniel J R, Maniar J L, Ganapati R 1984 An approach to leprosy work in South Bombay. Indian Journal of Leprosy 56: 280–291

Davey T F 1975 Common features in rapidly declining leprosy epidemics. Leprosy Review 46: 5–8

Georgiev C D, Kielstrup R W 1987 Blister calendar packs for the implementation of multiple drug therapy in DANIDA-assisted leprosy control projects in India. Leprosy Review 58: 249–255

Hamilton J 1983 Deformity prevention in the field: a systematic approach. Leprosy Review 54: 229–237

Huikeshoven H 1986 A simple urine spot test for monitoring dapsone self-administration in leprosy treatment. Bulletin of the World Health Organization, 64: 279–281

ILEP 1982 Leprosy control and primary health care. ILEP, London

Lechat M F, Vanderveken M 1983 Basic epidemiological indicators for monitoring leprosy control. Sasakawa Memorial Health Foundation, Tokyo

Legrange P H 1985 Strategy for leprosy control. International Journal of Leprosy 53: 278–288

Leprosy Review 1986 57: supplement 3. (Whole issue devoted to multidrug therapy)

Meade T W 1971 Epidemiology and Leprosy Control. Leprosy Review 42: 14–25

Nordeen S K 1969 Chemoprophylaxis in leprosy. Leprosy in India 41: 247–254

Ross W F 1987 A process for planning the introduction and implementation of multidrug therapy for leprosy. Leprosy Review 58: 313–323

Sansarricq H 1983 Recent changes in leprosy control. Leprosy Review special issue: 7S–16S

Skinsnes O K 1983 Epidemiology and decline of leprosy in Asia. International Journal of Dermatology 22: 348–367

World Health Organization 1988 A Guide to Leprosy Control. 2nd edn WHO, Geneva

Index